A Dad's Guide to Newborn Twins

A DAD'S GUIDE TO NEWBORN TWINS

TWINS

UNLEASH
YOUR INNER

SUPER
DAD

JENNIFER BONICELLI &
MEGHAN HERTZFELDT

Illustrations by James Olstein

R

ROCKRIDGE
PRESS

Interior and Cover Designer: Erik Jacobsen
Photo Art Director/Art Manager: Sara Feinstein
Editor: Mo Mozuch
Production Editor: Ashley Polikoff
Illustrations © 2020 James Olstein. Author photos courtesy of © Jenna Sparks Photography.

ISBN: Print 978-1-64739-128-7 | eBook 978-1-64739-129-4
R0

TO MATT AND JORDAN. WITHOUT YOU GUYS, NONE OF THIS WOULD HAVE BEEN POSSIBLE (WINK, WINK).

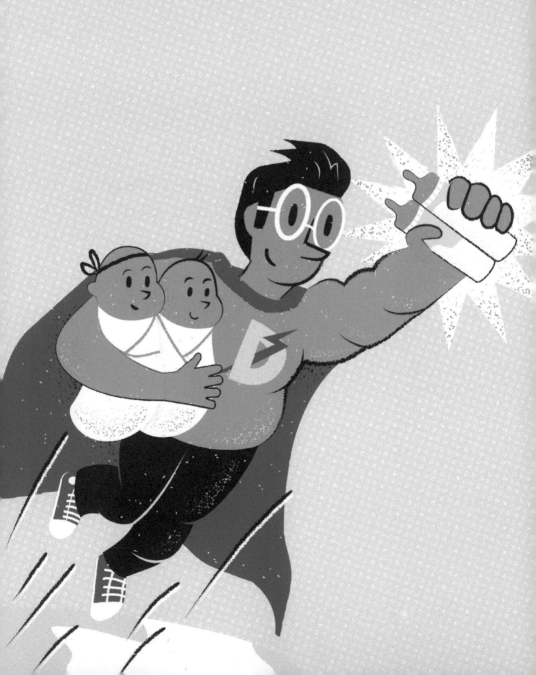

Table of Contents

Introduction

MAJOR CONGRATULATIONS ARE IN ORDER because you are about to become a dad to not one, but two babies. Bravo and welcome to a pretty unique group of multitasking overachievers: twin parents. The moment you see two heartbeats on an ultrasound will stick with you forever. Your life goes from zero to 60, suddenly, in one doctor's appointment. So whether you are still peeling your chin off the floor after your partner's doubly loaded announcement or you are clinking beers in celebration, you have come to the right place. There is no shortage of tips between the two of us and the men that stand beside us in our parenting journey. We can ensure you and your partner will be amply prepared for welcoming *two* babies. And while we can't predict what parenting hand you'll be dealt, we can teach you a thing or two about playing your cards.

You may be thinking, who are these two moms? What do they know about being a twin dad? We are Jenn and Meghan, the cofounders of the popular twin parenting blog *Two Came True* and coauthors of *You Can Two! The Essential Twins Preparation Guide*. Our careers in education helped our friendship flourish, but the real connection grew when our own twin parenting journeys began, first through infertility and then when we each had a set of fraternal twin boys. In comparing our experiences and turning to one another for guidance and advice, we found ourselves asking, "But what the hell do I do with *two*?" And so, our blog was born. It's a unique and welcoming online community, resource library, and inspirational outlet where twin parents can find the support and tools they need to thrive.

It wouldn't be fair if we took all of the credit because there are two men, the backbones of our families, who do things like put toothbrushes next to the kitchen sink during the newborn haze as a reminder to brush our teeth sometime before 2:00 p.m. They are the champions who are right beside us through every parenting mile-stone and challenge along the way. Every word written and all of the parenting advice we have crafted for this book has been created in conjunction with our husbands. Our journeys as two very different sets of twin parents, the wins and the epic fails, serve as the foundation for the twin parenting road map you hold in your hands.

Your new role as a family man, whether it be with a partner or as a single dad, is about to change . . . drastically. In this book, we keep it real. We give you a heads-up so you know what to expect, but also encourage you to embrace the messiness. Don't let the naysayers scare you: it's one heck of a ride with a lot to enjoy along the way.

Being a parent is learning to roll with the punches. As a parent of twins, well, you just have to nail that down a bit sooner. It's nice to have recommendations from others who have been in your shoes and understand that raising twins is a tricky situation. What we have chosen to share is a smattering of research, firsthand experience, and tips that have worked for our clients. If something we share just doesn't resonate, toss it out the window and try something new; there is no right or wrong approach to parenting.

Planning for one baby yet suddenly preparing to raise two can rock your world. So, as you sit with the wild news that you are expecting two (and maybe even begin to muddle through the stress of what is about to happen to your world), simply picking up this book is a step in the right direction. Your fatherly instincts will kick into gear, if they haven't already, and before you know it, you'll be headed to the hospital, with two infant car seats in your back seat ready to be filled. During the next few months, spend some time educating yourself. A little confidence goes a long way. You have what it takes to guide your growing family through this monumental first year.

Buckle up and enjoy the ride. Being a dad to twins is incredible!

How to Use this Book

We designed this book with the big picture in mind and the goal of preparing you for the entire journey—pregnancy, delivery, and surviving the first year with twins. There is so much to learn and do when expecting two, and this book is your crash course to help you prepare as much as possible before your babies arrive.

This book is an all-inclusive guide intended to be read soon after learning that your family is growing by four feet (instead of two) and then serve as a reference as you navigate each phase of "twinfancy." You'll find actionable guidance, personal anecdotes, checklists to keep you organized, and all the pertinent information you could possibly need through your partner's pregnancy and in your first year with twins.

Chapters 3 through 7 tackle the first year with your twins, including the ins and outs of doctor's appointments, developmental milestones, feeding, and sleeping tips, plus advice from us (and our partners). We want you to be able to refer back to these chapters to find any troubleshooting tools you will need when age-related challenges or questions arise.

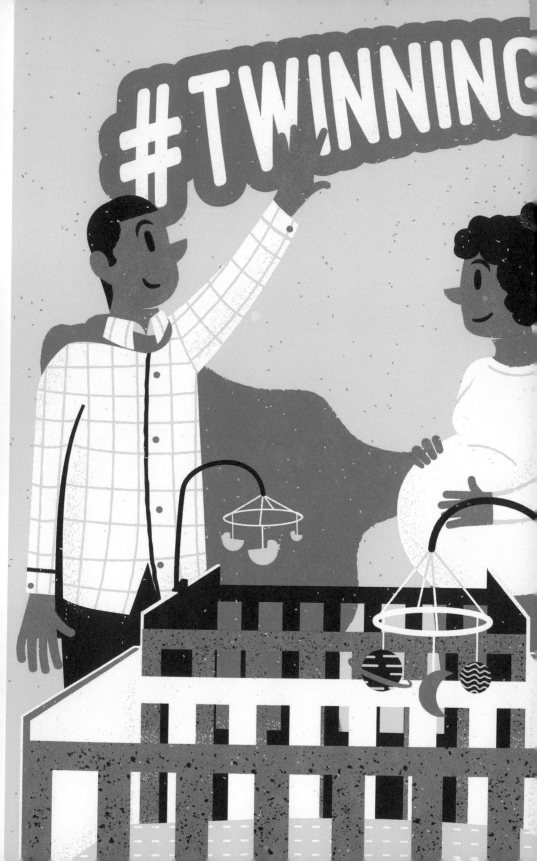

CHAPTER ONE

SUPPORTING YOUR PARTNER'S TWIN PREGNANCY

Think about life's greatest moments: unexpectedly winning a championship game, passing an exam you didn't study for, or scoring that first date with the person who ended up being your partner for life. Whatever they are will be distant memories the moment you become a twin dad. As you start to process how your life will change over the next several months, let us reassure you that you were made for this! Your twin parenting journey begins now, with this book. So, you can relax, you're off to a good start in your new role as *twin dad*.

There is plenty of information here for your first day on the job. We will guide you in supporting your partner throughout pregnancy and delivery, and diving into everything you need to know to be sure your home is baby ready. We cover the ins and outs of a potential (because not every twin parent experiences this) stay in the neonatal intensive care unit (NICU), and offer advice on baby gear and how to create a smart registry that helps you make important decisions as easily as possible.

"Are They Twins?"

Without fail, you will be asked this question about your twin babies by nearly every stranger you meet. Once you confirm that, yes, they are twins, you will be asked a second question: Are they identical or fraternal? (Yes, even parents who have boy/girl twins get this question.)

It's a question you had too (admit it) and the answer lies in biology.

Here's the short version. One fertilized egg splits, which means the one baby you planned on having becomes two. Identical twins, a monozygotic pregnancy, are about one-third of all twin pregnancies and come from one fertilized egg that splits into two embryos. Because these two embryos developed from one egg and one sperm, identical twins share the exact same DNA.

Fraternal twins are siblings that once shared a uterus. Fraternal twins, a dizygotic pregnancy, which make up two-thirds of all twin pregnancies, differ in that they are two babies from two separately fertilized eggs. They share a birthday but don't share the exact same DNA. Like any siblings, they share genetic traits inherited from their parents.

But wait, there's more! Twin pregnancies are further classified based on how the amniotic sac and placentas are divided. A fraternal twin pregnancy results in a dichorionic-diamniotic pregnancy, meaning your babies each have their own amniotic sac and placenta. Nobody has to share anything . . . yet.

In an identical twin pregnancy, the way an amniotic sac and placenta(s) are shared can be more complicated and will play a role in how your twin pregnancy is managed by your medical professional. Amboss, the medical learning platform, describes the following four types of twin pregnancies and the frequency with which they occur:

★ **Dichorionic-diamniotic.** Dichorionic-diamniotic pregnancies happen in about 20 to 30 percent of identical twin pregnancies. In this case, each fetus has its own individual amniotic sac and placenta.

★ **Monochorionic-diamniotic.** In monochorionic-diamniotic pregnancies, which account for the majority of twin pregnancies (about 70 percent), the fetuses have their own amniotic sacs but share a placenta.

★ **Monochorionic-monoamniotic.** In 1 to 5 percent of twin pregnancies, both the placenta and the amniotic sac are shared.

★ **Monochorionic-monoamniotic (conjoined twins).** In this type of twin pregnancy, the fetuses are conjoined and share both a placenta and the amniotic sac. These are rare, accounting for less than 0.01 percent of twin pregnancies.

Identical (monozygotic) twin pregnancies, where the placenta is shared, also include the risk of twin-to-twin transfusion syndrome (TTTS). We will discuss that in more depth later.

The medical jargon can be overwhelming, but remember that knowledge is power. Your role as dad and supportive partner requires you to be armed with all of this pertinent information as the doctor's appointments begin to fill your calendar.

Twin pregnancy is physically demanding and emotionally taxing. Because no two pregnancies are alike, it's hard to say exactly what your partner can expect. Your job is to uplift on the most challenging days and be a source of strength when the going gets tough. One of the most important roles you can play is acting as an advocate for your future family-to-be.

Surrogacy

Parenthood is a wonderful gift. Thanks to surrogacy, many more people (couples and single parents alike) get to experience it. Making the decision to use a surrogate, and whom you choose to be your gestational carrier, are very personal, private, and complicated choices. Traditional surrogacy involves artificially inseminating the surrogate, who carries the baby, with the father's sperm. A gestational surrogate, generally a more common route taken in the United States, becomes pregnant via in vitro fertilization (IVF) with an egg from the mother (or via an egg donor) and the father's sperm.

Bryce and Jeffrey Abplanalp-Wright
@growingupwithdads

We knew we wanted to be parents and have our own family. That's what initially drew us together as a couple. We weren't sure that was possible, being gay . . . We started our family through surrogacy. Living in a very conservative and religious state, we had some challenges finding a surrogate who was willing to work with a same-sex couple.

We finally "matched" with our amazing angel of a surrogate and transferred two embryos—Bryce biologically connected to one and Jeffrey to the other. Our twin pregnancy was fairly uneventful and standard. We attended the vast majority of appointments and ultrasounds with our surrogate and met at least weekly for lunch or just to hang out. After not knowing each other prior to our journey, we became fast friends. Right around the 34-week mark we got the call of our lives. Like all parents, we were a bundle of emotions and couldn't believe the day had finally arrived. By this point we had created an unbreakable bond with our surrogate and regarded her as nothing short of a hero. On that day, she labored and delivered twins through an unmedicated birth. On November 27, Larue (Rue) and Ridge were born. They were premature and weren't quite ready to take on the world alone. Our twins spent about two weeks in the NICU learning how to breathe and eat on their own, but in the end, we're now a happy family of four.

The Medical Team

Early on, two of the big decisions you'll need to make are selecting the medical team that will be in charge of your partner's pregnancy and where this whole affair will go down. Because you are having twins, you need to do a little extra research on hospitals beforehand because those decisions will have consequences down the road if complications arise.

PICKING THE RIGHT DOCTOR

Choosing the person or practice that will deliver your twin babies is a monumental decision. While the final decision will mostly lie with your partner, you will play a big role in helping evaluate her needs and manage her health care. As a couple expecting twins, you will both spend quite a bit of time with this person, more so than in singleton pregnancies. So, while it is important that your partner is comfortable with the doctor, this person will be guiding both of you into parenthood, which is why you also need to trust the person and medical practice involved.

You should ask thoughtful questions and look into your insurance policy. Insurance often plays a role in the doctors you are able to choose. When picking the doctor to deliver your twins, consider the following:

★ What is the doctor's experience in delivering twins?

★ Is the doctor a part of a medical group or do they practice alone?

★ How does the OB/practice handle delivery day? Who will deliver the babies if your chosen doctor isn't available?

★ Does your doctor perform sonograms in the office? If they don't you will be making additional trips to medical offices for frequent ultra-sounds.

★ Is the doctor you love affiliated with your preferred hospital? Does the hospital have a NICU?

★ Is the office location convenient to your work and home?

★ Many doctors deliver twins at 38 weeks. What is the doctor's policy on this?

★ What is the doctor's policy on delivering twins? Is a vaginal delivery possible or do they only perform C-sections for multiple births? If you can deliver vaginally, will it be in an operating room (OR) in case complications arise?

★ How does the doctor manage pain during delivery? Oftentimes epidurals are strongly encouraged in case an emergency C-section is needed for one or both of your babies.

PICKING THE RIGHT HOSPITAL

Choosing the doctor to deliver your twins and the hospital at which you want to deliver go hand in hand. First, check to make sure your preferred hospital is covered by your insurance. Then narrow down your choices to hospitals that have a NICU on campus. Finally, under-stand the level of care a NICU can provide, because they really do vary quite a bit.

Meghan: When I started researching hospitals, my hormonal head was all over the place. I was making it complicated. My hus-band jumped in and simplified the search for us. After consulting our insurance coverage, we weighed two major factors for each hospital: the NICU and how close it was to our house. We chose a hospital that was small and intimate. It had a great NICU and happened to be connected to our doctor's office, which was a huge perk toward the end of our pregnancy. I ended up walking across the hall for weekly NSTs (fetal non-stress tests) after my appointments and it made life much easier, especially when walking wasn't.

According to the March of Dimes, there are four levels of NICU care, ranging from basic care all the way to surgical subspecialties and on-site anesthesiologists. In most cases, babies who are admitted to the NICU are born before 37 weeks, have low birth weight, or are born with a medical condition (including trouble breathing, heart conditions, infections, or birth defects).

LEVEL I. They provide basic care for healthy, full-term babies. These units will also stabilize near-term babies so they can be transferred to specialized facilities.

LEVEL II. Advanced care units care for babies born at 32 weeks or later, or for babies who are recovering from serious medical conditions.

LEVEL III. Specialized care units provide care for babies born earlier than 32 weeks or born with a critical illness. These units staff pediatric specialists and provide respiratory support.

LEVEL IV. These units provide the highest level of neonatal care in hospitals with pediatric surgeons and anesthesiologists on staff.

The reality is multiple births have a higher chance of a NICU stay than singleton pregnancies. You'll want to try to eliminate the scenario where you're assisting in your partner's recovery at one hospital and traveling across town to another hospital to be with your babies in a NICU.

Here are some other things to consider while you are preparing to deliver twins:

★ What is the hospital's policy on where women expecting multiples give birth? It isn't uncommon for multiples to be delivered vaginally, in an OR as a precaution.

★ Is an anesthesiologist available 24 hours a day? It's nice to know ahead of time if there will always be someone at the hospital to assist in an emergency C-section.

★ What is the hospital's nurse-to-mom ratio? The fewer moms each nurse has to care for, the better.

★ Who is allowed to be in the room during delivery? Some expectant parents want the entire family to be a part of the birth, while others want privacy. Be aware that multiple births are complicated and require extra medical personnel in the room.

★ How far is the hospital from your house and/or your workplace? You will be the one driving to the hospital, and while you won't be able to control the traffic on D-Day, you can control how far you are driving.

When to See the Perinatologist

Perinatologists are maternal-fetal medicine specialists in charge of caring for fetuses in high-risk pregnancies. They usually come into the picture when a pregnancy turns high risk due to medical conditions that develop, like birth defects in utero, gestational diabetes, preeclampsia, or problems with fetal growth, to name a few. However, some women will be referred before becoming pregnant or early in pregnancy if they have a history of pregnancy loss, obesity, advanced maternal age, or health conditions like diabetes, lupus, or blood or endocrine issues.

As a part of your medical team, a perinatologist will work with your OB and other pertinent medical professionals to be sure the outcome of your twin pregnancy is the best possible. Perinatologists, in some cases, might be with you for a short while, monitoring your pregnancy; in other cases they might be a part of your medical team for the duration of the pregnancy.

Meghan: *I was referred to a perinatologist because extra fluid was found in Baby B's amniotic sac. I will never forget the look on my husband's face: he looked like a deer in headlights. I could see the wheels turning in his head as we realized things might not go as smoothly as we had hoped. This was one of the first moments in our pregnancy where we felt completely out of control.*

We felt a little uneasy because we weren't sure if everything was going to be okay. One appointment with a specialist later and we could take a deep breath. We realized having to see a specialized doc had its perks. Not only were the boys being closely monitored, we had all of the questions that were keeping us up at night answered, and we got to see our babies on the big screen even more.

Jenn: *A routine ultrasound appointment took a turn when an echogenic intracardiac focus was found on each of our babies' hearts. These small deposits of calcium collect in the muscles of a baby's heart [and] usually go away in the third trimester. Because they can be associated with chromosomal problems in babies, we began seeing a perinatologist as well as our OB for the remainder of my pregnancy. Hearing that something might be wrong with your babies is worrisome, but the additional appointments helped reassure us and put our minds at ease.*

Rest and Nutrition

It's no secret that pregnancy is hard; growing tiny humans—two for that matter—is physically and emotionally demanding. Your partner will experience physical changes at a pretty rapid pace: the belly, the boobs, the hormones. (Oh, the hormones.)

As the old saying goes, "Mom takes care of the baby; dad takes care of the mom." We cannot emphasize enough that your role as dad is to recognize and advocate for her needs, especially when she struggles. There will be times where she is mentally drained, physically taxed, or swimming in the fog of sleep deprivation. In those moments, the greatest gift you can give her is meeting a need she didn't even know she had.

Your pregnant partner doesn't want to slow down until she has to. Nine months go by fast and she has a lot to accomplish in that short time. However, the one thing a twin-mom-to-be should avoid is overdoing it. Swollen feet and a belly that's growing by the minute bring on debilitating aches and pains. Don't be surprised if you are taxed with helping her out of bed at night so she can pee . . . many, many times. This is your time to shine. Show her how you can make life easier when the going gets tough. Maintaining a restful schedule and a healthy diet are crucial for her to have a healthy pregnancy.

HOW MANY CALORIES?

There is some truth to the cliché that your partner is "eating for three," so when mom is slamming an extra taco it's probably not the time for any wisecracks. Be supportive. Let the lady eat!

Growing two babies is hard work. However, healthy weight gain with a twin pregnancy is incredibly important. Additional healthy calories must be added to your partner's typical diet. For a woman carrying twins, the American College of Obstetrics and Gynecology suggests adding 600 calories per day to her usual diet, but this can vary depending on her prepregnancy weight.

Pregnancy weight gain is highly dependent on each person and her prepregnancy body mass index (BMI). According to the Institute of Medicine (now the National Academy of Medicine), women carrying twins should gain:

★ 37 to 54 pounds if their BMI is 18.5 to 24.9

★ 31 to 50 pounds if their BMI is 25 to 29.9

★ 25 to 42 pounds if their BMI is higher than 30

What does this have to do with you? Well, you can ensure the meals you eat together are packed with nutritious calories (The Institute of Medicine suggests 20 to 25 percent protein, 45 to 50 percent carbs, and 30 percent fats) and her purse is filled with protein-dense snacks. Don't be surprised if she asks for the occasional Italian sub at midnight, either. (Yes, you have to go get it.)

It's not uncommon for pregnant women to struggle with nausea or not feel hungry. Sometimes she may need gentle reminders to grab a snack, ensuring that she is getting the extra calories her body needs to nourish your growing babies.

Meghan: My husband was a key player in helping me get my diet back on track after I discovered I'd gained 12 pounds in one week during a routine checkup! He didn't know whether to laugh or to be concerned when the doctor told us the news. It turns out I was a little heavy on my fruit intake that week and I needed to dial down my sugar consumption. I am thankful my husband was dedicated to coming to appointments when he could because I felt especially defeated that day. Having a wingman at each appointment gave me the comfort and support I needed when twin pregnancy got tough.

Jenn: My pregnancy was nausea-ridden from the get-go and I began vomiting daily from 16 to 36 weeks. Having an appetite was difficult mainly because I couldn't even open our refrigerator without getting sick. My husband played an essential role in helping me keep enough calories in my body to gain weight. He got creative in the kitchen and helped me find a few foods I could keep down or reminded me to try to eat, even when I resisted. He was the one person that did whatever he could to ease the misery of the weeks I spent nauseated and vomiting.

VITAMINS AND NUTRIENTS EVERY PREGNANT PARTNER NEEDS

Nutrition is one of the key players in having a healthy pregnancy. Here's the breakdown of essential vitamins and nutrients that are crucial for a healthy pregnancy, according to the American Pregnancy

Association. As always, chat with your doctor about your partner's specific needs.

ZINC

Zinc is essential for normal immune function and when taken during pregnancy will help lower the risk of preterm birth due to maternal infections. The recommended dose is 30 milligrams per day. Foods include breakfast cereal, hummus, dark chocolate, crab, and lobster.

FOLIC ACID

Six hundred micrograms of folic acid daily before and during pregnancy help prevent birth defects that affect your baby's brain and spinal cord. Foods include dark leafy greens (spinach and kale), citrus fruit, lentils, eggs, and broccoli.

CALCIUM

Pregnant women should aim to get 1,500 milligrams of calcium per day to help the development of your babies' musculoskeletal, nervous, and circulatory systems. Calcium also helps lower the risk of developing preeclampsia. Foods include dairy, white beans, and broccoli.

IRON

Women carrying twins are at a higher risk of developing anemia, which can cause low birth weight. Pregnant women need about 30 milligrams of iron daily to help reduce their risk of hypertension. Foods include shellfish, spinach, and dark chocolate.

MAGNESIUM

Magnesium can help reduce fetal growth restriction and preeclampsia, and increase birth weight. It also helps strengthen your baby's bones and teeth and aids in the development of their central nervous system. Pregnant women should get 98 milligrams per day by eating foods like avocados, bananas, and whole grains.

VITAMIN D

On average, prenatal vitamins contain 400 IU of vitamin D. Studies have shown that women who take 4,000 IU of vitamin D daily can prevent preterm labor, premature birth, and infections. Aside from getting outside often, women should focus on eating foods like fatty fish, milk, and fortified orange juice.

WATER

Staying hydrated is essential in pregnancy. Water plays an important role in healthy fetal development. Water helps form the placenta and the amniotic sac during pregnancy. Pregnant women should aim to drink 8 to 12 (8-ounce) glasses of water a day.

COMMON COMPLICATIONS

By this point, you are aware that twin pregnancies have a higher risk of complications. This doesn't necessarily mean any of these complications will happen to your partner, and we aren't sharing common complications to add more stress to your plate, but remember what we said earlier . . . knowledge is power. According to Children's Wisconsin, here are some complications you may encounter:

AMNIOTIC FLUID ISSUES. Amniotic fluid surrounds your babies in the womb and aids in the development of their muscles, lungs, and digestive systems. Amniotic fluid levels are measured during each ultrasound. Low amniotic levels early in pregnancy can signify growth problems, while low levels later in pregnancy may be a sign of placental failure. High levels aren't usually problematic but can put your partner at higher risk for growth problems or premature birth.

ANEMIA. Anemia in pregnancy is associated with low birth weight, premature birth, and maternal mortality. Anemia describes a condition where there are not enough healthy red blood cells to carry oxygen to tissue in the body. Pregnant women develop anemia because their bodies are producing an excess of blood to bring nutrients to the baby. Generally it is a mild condition, but if left untreated it can become more serious. Iron or vitamin supplements are generally prescribed for anemia in pregnancy.

CORD ENTANGLEMENT. Cord entanglement happens in almost all monoamniotic-monochorionic twin pregnancies where both babies share an amniotic sac and a placenta. Although they share a placenta, they have separate umbilical cords, which inevitably will tangle thanks to the absence of an amniotic membrane to separate them. Cord entanglement can hinder fetal movement and development. In many cases of cord entanglement, doctors may want to deliver as soon as the babies are developed enough to survive (around 24 weeks) and may require that your pregnancy is monitored in the hospital.

C-SECTION DELIVERY. There is very little research available to clearly guide families expecting twins in the optimal method of delivery. You need to clearly understand the benefits and risks of a vaginal delivery of your twins, as well as those of a C-section delivery. According to WhatToExpect.com, the method of delivery will often depend on how both babies are positioned, how the baby closest to the cervix is positioned, how Baby B is positioned (especially after Baby A is delivered), whether you have one placenta or two during the pregnancy, and whether your twins are similar in size.

TWIN-TO-TWIN TRANSFUSION SYNDROME (TTTS). Johns Hopkins describes TTTS as a complication in monozygotic-monochorionic identical twin pregnancies. An imbalance in the blood exchange between twins causes one twin to give away more blood than it receives. The donor twin suffers from malnourishment and organ failure, and the recipient twin has too much blood and can develop cardiac complications. A minimally invasive surgery can correct the imbalance and offers families the best chance of having two healthy babies.

POSTPARTUM HEMORRHAGE. Postpartum hemorrhage is excessive bleeding after the birth of a baby, most commonly after a C-section. While it usually occurs immediately after birth, it can happen later as well. Hemorrhage is characterized by uncontrolled bleeding, decrease in blood pressure and red blood cell count, increased heart rate or swelling, and pain in vaginal tissues.

BED REST BLUES

It is a common misconception that twin pregnancy and restrictive bed rest go hand in hand. Just because one is expecting multiples doesn't mean she is destined for bed rest. Bed rest can range from lightening up her daily activity to being completely confined to the couch or a hospital bed.

Regardless of what type of limitations your partner is prescribed, we strongly suggest that you and your partner have a detailed conversation with your OB about why bed rest is recommended and what the prescription is aiming to remedy in the pregnancy. Bed rest limits your partner's ability to work and participate in your daily lives. It can become a profound hardship.

Should your partner experience some sort of modified bed rest or hospital bed rest, you may find the following bits of advice, gathered from families who were impacted by activity restriction during their pregnancy, helpful. As the supportive man in your bedridden partner's life, your workload will feel heavier. Cooking, cleaning, working full-time, and taking care of any other children (or fur babies) now falls on your shoulders. Here's how you'll manage:

NURTURE YOUR RELATIONSHIP. While she is confined to your house or a hospital, you both won't be able to enjoy the usual nights out that are so crucial to your relationship. When you can, find ways to bring a date night to her. Maybe it's making her a cup of tea and snuggling on the couch to watch her favorite rom-com or bringing home takeout from your favorite date-night spot.

FIND SUPPORT. It takes a village, fellas. You cannot be her sole support. Be sure she has plenty of visitors and introduce her to Sidelines .org, where she can find a community of women experiencing high-risk pregnancies and bed rest.

Gestational Diabetes

Gestational diabetes is one of those pregnancy terms that makes expectant women everywhere uneasy. Sitting around a doctor's office drinking sugary drinks and waiting to have your blood drawn is cringe-worthy.

The Centers for Disease Control and Prevention (CDC) describes gestational diabetes as a type of diabetes found in women who have not previously been diagnosed with the condition prior to pregnancy. Women expecting twins are at a higher risk for developing this condition. Typically it shows up during the middle of pregnancy, which is why a pregnant woman will be tested within the 24-to-28-week mark. Her blood will be drawn after fasting and then again after drinking a sugary solution. Additional testing may be required if her blood sugar levels are high after drinking the solution.

Generally speaking, pregnant women do not experience symptoms before they learn they have gestational diabetes. Occasionally women will experience fatigue, nausea, unusual thirst, or frequent bladder infections. It's important for expectant moms to stay on top of regular prenatal appointments, exercise throughout pregnancy, deal with any excess weight before getting pregnant, and ensure the majority of calories come from foods that are nutrient rich and low in processed sugars.

If your pregnant partner does end up with gestational diabetes, rest assured the condition can generally be managed with diet and exercise, and if necessary, with medication. She will be required to frequently (daily) check her blood sugar levels and monitor her urine for ketones. You both can expect her blood sugar levels to return to normal shortly after delivery, but you should know that she will be at a higher risk for developing type 2 diabetes as a result. Continual monitoring and responsible health care will be necessary for her future health and pregnancies.

ENTERTAINMENT. Binge-watching only goes so far. Reach out to friends to gather books or teach her a new hobby that will help keep her entertained. Adult coloring books, fluffy blankets, heck, even creative toys like a Lite-Brite are fun items for a woman confined to her bed.

Your partner will be relying on everyone else to meet her basic needs. She will be uncomfortable and physically limited, but don't downplay how challenging bed rest will be for you either. This too shall pass. The time your partner spends on bed rest will feel like a blip in the grand scheme of things.

Make sure you find time to meet your personal needs. Let go of the guilt. Snag a beer with a friend or go to the range to hit some balls. Recharging is crucial and okay because your mental health is equally as important during this time. If you aren't doing well, you won't be able to stay positive around your partner and she'll feed off that. If she's struggling, she will need to rely on you to help her work through it. Communicating and connecting now will only make you a stronger team once your babies are here.

Nursery and Baby Gear

Although you're expecting two, there is actually very little you need in duplicate. Before you drain your bank account in an unnecessary shopping spree, remember that less is more when expecting twins.

Begin by collecting hand-me-downs. Next, scour garage sales because babies grow quickly and there is always a mind-blowing amount of stuff that never gets used. When you find your nursery closet full of unopened diapers and clothes with tags still attached, consider returning and exchanging these items for things you need.

While your twins are temporary tenants of your partner or surrogate's uterus, most of your job is being emotionally supportive and attentive. Researching baby gear, planning your nursery, and beginning to assemble things is an area where you can have a tangible impact.

These things take time and preparation. With the simple guidance included in this section, you will be able to successfully tackle this part of your baby preparation and help ease the stress your partner might be feeling about getting your lives and home ready for two babies.

Two Kids, One Nursery

They may be pint-size, but man can they take up a lot of space. Down the road you may separate your twins into their own rooms, but in our experience, families expecting twins plan one nursery for both of their babies to share. For most, the challenge becomes fitting all the nursery essentials into a limited space. Regardless of the setup you have, you will need *two* cribs. Yes, crib sharing is a common practice for twin parents, but eventually babies learn to roll and sit up so they need their own safe space to sleep. Arrange the cribs in the nursery, ideally on separate walls or at least with enough space in between for you to move around. Beyond that, you can get by with the basics, like a rocker, a changing table, and maybe a bookshelf or some baskets with toys.

Have fun creating the space of your dreams! You get to put your personal touch on what is to become one of the most important rooms in your house. The nursery projects help you, Dad, feel more connected to the pregnancy, something that won't be an issue for your partner (the babies aren't living in *your* uterus after all).

THE BIG LIST

Look no further! Here is the only baby registry cheat sheet you will need. Between shower gifts, hand-me-downs, and a little of your own shopping, you'll be ready with all the must-haves when you bring your twins home from the hospital. When in doubt, keep those tags attached and the receipts in an envelope. As your babies get older, you can adjust your stockpile based on what you did and did not use.

BABY BASICS

★ Burp cloths

★ Diaper cream

★ Diapers and wipes (buy a variety of sizes)

★ Gas drops

★ Gripe water

★ Hats

★ Infant first-aid kit

★ Lotion

★ Baby Nasal Aspirator, aka "snotsuckers"

★ Onesies (We recommend onesies with zippers rather than buttons. Also, buying onesies with feet eliminates the need for those baby socks that never stay on.)

★ Pacifiers and travel straps (lots)

★ Swaddles or receiving blankets

★ Thermometer

NURSERY ESSENTIALS

★ Baskets to organize clothes and diapers

★ Bassinets (2) (Incline sleepers are no longer recommended by the American Academy of Pediatrics.)

★ Blackout shades

★ Changing table (1)

★ Changing table pad (1)

* Clock (You want something you can see in the dark to help track feedings and wake times so you can eventually get your babies on a schedule.)

* Cribs and mattresses (2)

* Crib sheets (2 to 3 sets)

* Diaper pail. (Preferably one like Ubbi makes that use regular garbage bags.)

* Hamper

* Humidifier

* Lamp

* Playpen or portable playard (1 to 2)

* Rocking chair or glider (1)

* Side table

* Video monitor (Buy one that has two cameras and a split screen.)

* Waterproof mattress pads (4 to 6)

* White noise machine

BATH TIME

* Baby bath sling (we like the ones made with mesh), sink insert, or infant tub

* Bath thermometer

* Bath toys

* Bathtub mat

* Faucet guard

* Infant washcloths

* ★ Knee pad (You'll thank us when you're on your knees bending over the tub.)

* ★ Towels

TOYS AND FUN STUFF

Ahh, toys. A blessing and a curse for expectant twin parents. If you can score hand-me-downs in this department, do it. When you need to invest, maybe get some of the larger items like playmats, saucers, bouncers, or swings. Only buy the basics and rotate your babies in and out of each. One of your babies might love one contraption but despise another. Remember, less is more.

* ★ Bouncer (1)

* ★ Baby activity saucer or activity center (1)

* ★ Lovies or small stuffed animals

* ★ Playmat (1 to 2)

* ★ Rattles or noisemakers

* ★ Stroller/car seat toys

* ★ Swing (1)

TRAVEL GEAR

Getting out of the house with two babies in tow is going to require you to channel your inner survivalist. Why? You'll want to be prepared for anything, ready to tackle the most unexpected scenario that might come your way with all necessary essentials in one bag with easy-to-access pockets.

* ★ Baby carriers (2) or a twin-specific carrier

* ★ Car seat covers (Nursing covers double well for this purpose.)

* ★ Car seat mirrors (2)

* ★ Car seats (2)

* ★ Double stroller that accommodates two car seats

* ★ Diaper backpack

* ★ Portable changing mat

FEEDING

Whether your partner chooses to breastfeed, pump, use formula, or some combination of it all, you'll want to take an all-hands-on-deck approach. Think of your partner as the quarterback and you're the offensive line. Though you can't physically breastfeed, the extra set of hands and your supportive nature are what your partner needs most. You can help position the babies when your partner is tandem breastfeeding or bottle-feed one baby while your partner feeds the other. Stay calm, be patient, and remember your job is to lower her anxiety, not increase it.

* ★ Nursing pillows such as Boppy (2) or TwinZ Pillow (1)

* ★ Bottle brush

* ★ Bottle drying rack

* ★ Bottles and nipples

* ★ Bottle soap

* ★ Breast pump (Many models are covered by insurance.)

* ★ Formula mixing pitcher

* ★ Extra set of pump parts (Have the nurses properly fit your partner at the hospital for the correct size.)

* ★ High chairs (2) (You won't need high chairs immediately, but down the road when your babies start eating solids, you will need them. Our space-saving suggestion is to invest in the lobster claw–style seats that attach to tabletops or counters.)

★ Microwave sterilizer bags for cleaning pumps and bottles

★ Nursing bras or tank tops

Stroller

You will use your stroller often, and ideally you'll have it for years. And there are probably what feels like billions of stroller options to choose from, so how do you decide? Are you a city slicker who needs something compact? Are you an outdoorsy family in need of off-roading tires? There are strollers to fit every need.

Twin families can choose from in-line, side-by-side, or convertible strollers. In-line models offer parents the ability to sit two babies one in front of the other, without doubling the width of a single stroller. They are slightly harder to maneuver and often don't offer the same space or amenities for both seats. Side-by-side models are easier to maneuver but their width can make doorways, elevators, or jamming it in the back of your car a challenge. Convertible strollers are usually great investments for growing families. Starting as a single stroller, additional seats (up to three total seats for some models) can be added.

Just like when buying a new car, you will want to test out your babies' new ride. Take it for a spin around the store, trying to maneuver a variety of double stroller configurations around and through doorways. Bring a measuring tape and a notebook with you to jot down dimensions. How small is it when it's collapsed? Can it fit in the back of your car? Does it easily fold, maybe even with one hand? Does it accommodate two infant car seats? What is the rider weight limit (in case you need to accommodate older children too)? Think about the places you go most often and how a particular stroller will serve your needs.

We often hear from our clients that just one double stroller doesn't cut it and they end up investing in things like infant car seat strollers, where two car seats can easily snap in for things like running quick errands around town, or single umbrella strollers when parents split for the day to divide and conquer.

Strollers, especially when you buy multiple styles, may set you back a bit. The good news is that the secondhand market for strollers is hot. You might be able to find a gently used version of the one you want that's outside your budget. Or if you buy new, know you'll get a bit of your investment back when it's time to retire this must-have baby gear.

Car Seat

Like strollers, there are countless types of car seats to choose from. The choices include infant rear-facing car seats, convertible models, 3-in-1 car seats, and booster seats. According to the American Academy of Pediatrics, car seats are a permanent fixture in your life until your kids are 57 inches tall or 12 years old, which may impact the car seat model you choose. Infant car seats, the ones with the handles that you can carry around, are rear-facing and intended for use with infants up to about 30 pounds. Convertible seats can switch from rear-facing to forward-facing when your kids are old enough to turn around (two years of age at the earliest). The 3-in-1 option grows with your child until they need to transition to a booster seat at 40 pounds. Finally, booster seats elevate your children in the car to ensure the seat belt appropriately sits across their body. Just be sure that your child fits the height and weight guidelines required for the particular seat you use.

As you consider which car seat brand and model will work best, we encourage you to look at pricing, popularity, and how it fits in your car *after* you have carefully researched safety ratings. All car seats sold today have to meet the safety standards set forth by the National Highway Traffic Safety Administration; however, it is a good idea to ensure that the seat you choose has additional side impact protection and additionally meets the American Academy of Pediatrics recommendations. Beyond that, discuss these questions with your partner:

How long do we intend to use the car seat?

What are our plans for our family? Will we have more children who will need infant seats?

What space does our back seat provide? Measure the car against the dimensions of the car seat. You'll be shocked how small your car can become once you install two infant car seats.

Do we want to have more than one set of seats for a second car? Budget and convertibility may be of importance here.

How often will we be moving the seat in and out of the car? Consider the footprint, weight of the seat, and ease of installation.

Do we want to use the seats with a stroller? If so, find ones as part of a travel system or a universal car seat stroller like a Snap-N-Go to use until the twins outgrow their infant seats.

Car seats have a lingo all their own. This glossary from CarSeat.org will help you understand the safety systems and accessories for the particular seat you choose.

★ **Adjustable foot.** This system allows you to adjust a rear-facing seat to the correct angle.

★ **Automated locking.** This feature locks the seat belt into a set position, holding the passenger or car seat in place during a crash.

★ **Best positioning booster.** This is a type of booster seat that uses built-in belt guides to appropriately position the vehicle's seat belt on your child.

★ **Belt path.** A seat belt will thread through the car seat through belt paths. Typically there are separate paths for rear-facing and forward-facing positioning.

★ **Chest clip.** This is the buckle that sits across your child's chest. It should be positioned at armpit level.

★ **Detachable base.** This base for a rear-facing infant seat keeps the car seat secure, allowing you to lock the seat into the base and easily unlatch it from the base when you're ready to go.

★ **Expiration.** Car seats expire after six years. If you inherit a seat or grab one secondhand, be sure to find the expiration date located on the manufacturer label (either on the sides or base of the seat). It's not possible to verify a crash history with car seat manufacturers, so this is one area where you want to set the bar high.

★ **Level indicator.** This feature is a level embedded into the car seat that allows you to adjust the seat correctly. Follow the guidelines on the side of the seat to ensure your seat is at the proper angle for your baby.

★ **LATCH system.** The Lower Anchors and Tethers for Children system is found in cars manufactured after 2002 and is designed to make car seat installation easier without having to use vehicle belts.

★ **Lower anchors.** Bars embedded in your back seat that provide latching security for your car seat

★ **Lower anchor attachments.** These attachments on the car seat are used to secure the seat in the vehicle without the use of the vehicle seat belt.

★ **Recalls.** Check with the manufacturer regularly to be sure there aren't recalls for your particular car seat model.

★ **Registration.** Each car seat comes with a registration card that you can fill out and return with your contact information so that you will be promptly notified of recalls.

★ **Tether.** A tether strap and hood system anchors the top of a forward-facing car seat to an anchor behind the passenger seats in a car.

Cribs

Yes, your babies will eventually need separate cribs. The professionals encourage families to carefully reconsider crib sharing due to the risk of sudden infant death syndrome, or SIDS. There is a plethora of sleeping solutions on the market today, including cribs, bassinets, Pack 'n Plays, and floor mattresses. Going with our less-is-more philosophy, we like to encourage families to purchase baby gear with longevity in mind.

Our sleeping contraption of choice is a convertible crib, which converts from an infant crib to a toddler bed and into a twin bed or sometimes even a double bed. The initial investment may sting a little, but ultimately this is a purchase that will serve your family well into the future.

As your twins develop their sleep habits over the first few years of their life, your sleeping arrangements may need to adapt. We'll dive into sleep training later, but while we're on the subject of baby gear, consider snagging something portable, like a playpen or playard, to help manage the sleep challenges that lie ahead.

The Handyman?

Your newborn twins won't come with a manual, but all the crap you have to buy for them does! Sadly, most baby gear doesn't come ready to use right out of the box. In most cases some assembly is required. Cribs, strollers, shelving, and car seats need to be assembled or properly installed, requiring you to know your way around a power tool.

We know that not every expectant dad is proficient in furniture assembly, which is why society invented YouTube. Whether you are the type to strap on a tool belt and get down to business or you're scouring Angie's List in a desperate search for a handyman, remember that the Internet is filled with videos that can serve as step-by-step visual instruction manuals for your assembly needs. Search by brands and model numbers for specific instructions. You can always invite a few buddies over for beers and put them to work! It's kind of like moving in to your college dorm, but, you know, for babies.

Most companies offer installation services, online instruction manuals, and helpful hotlines to call for questions and problems with broken or missing parts. For things like car seat installations visit SafeKids.org to find car seat checkup events or installation stations near your home.

Whether you're going the do-it-yourself route or choosing to hire out, rest assured that resources are available to help you get all of the baby gear assembled well in advance of your impending delivery. Word to the wise: don't leave this to the last minute. Twins have been known to make their appearance earlier than expected.

Trimester Checklists

Not only does Santa make a list and check it twice, so does a well-prepared twin dad. Twin pregnancy may seem like it takes forever, but the end sneaks up on you. Here's a trimester-specific list filled with practical and personal reminders to help you prepare, both physically and mentally, for when your newborn twins arrive.

FIRST TRIMESTER

The first trimester will be a whirlwind of doctor's appointments and, for your partner, physical changes. It will be harder to hide a twin pregnancy because of her rapidly growing belly so word might get out sooner than you expected.

★ Plan your twin pregnancy announcement.

★ Share the news with your loved ones, either privately or publicly, when you are both ready.

★ Understand your health insurance and what it covers. Research and decide on hospitals and doctors.

★ Begin discussing your vision for the nursery so you can save if you have larger projects in mind.

★ Research paternity leave and discuss time off with your employer.

★ Research Family and Medical Leave Act (FMLA) paperwork and paternity leave options.

★ Review and adjust your finances to prepare for how pregnancy and maternity/paternity leave will affect your bottom line.

★ If possible, set up accounts for your babies' future and education. At the very least, get life insurance.

SECOND TRIMESTER

During these short months, your partner is probably feeling better than ever, which means you are too. Live it up! Go on dates while you can, take a trip, remain social! This is the time to really enjoy the ride.

★ Begin researching child care options.

★ Research baby gear brands and create a baby registry.

★ Research hospital and pediatrician options. Start scheduling tours of any birthing facilities you may be considering.

★ Begin taking parenting classes that spark your interest (infant CPR, etc.).

★ Begin projects in your nursery.

★ Begin to assemble nursery furniture.

★ Go on a babymoon.

★ Have a baby shower.

★ If applicable, adjust your estate planning to include your future children. Be sure to address your children's inheritance and guardianship.

THIRD TRIMESTER

This final stretch can be a pretty unpredictable time in a twin pregnancy. The hope is for a full-term delivery, but just in case that's not in your cards, it's wise to get as much done as you can, sooner rather than later.

★ Create a birth plan with your partner.

★ Soak up last-minute date nights.

★ Prep some freezer meals.

★ Research, interview, and decide on a pediatrician.

★ Finalize your hospital choice and preregister.

★ Finalize nursery organization and wash clothes and sheets.

★ Pack hospital bags.

★ Have car seats installed and checked by a professional.

★ Establish a communication chain so that all your family and friends can be notified when your babies arrive.

★ Cook and freeze meals to have on hand throughout those weeks and months after delivery.

★ Temperature check: Ask your partner how they are doing. Communication is key to your relationship. You want to make sure you're rock-solid before these babies arrive. You both are going through a lot. A quick check-in with each other goes a long way.

Six Signs of Early Labor

Speaking from experience, you may end up in the hospital ready to meet your twin babies only to find out that your partner's water didn't break, she just peed her pants. Since twin pregnancies are at a higher risk for preterm labor, both you *and* your partner need to know the signs of early labor. Doctors get a lot of calls from expectant parents with all kinds of questions. Your doctor would rather you call with 15 false alarms than wait too long and be faced with something more serious. While preterm labor does not always result in premature birth, the earlier the complication is addressed, the better the outcome for mom and the babies. Here's what the American Pregnancy Association advises pregnant women to look for:

1. **Vaginal discharge.** An increase or change (watery, mucus-like, or bloody) in her vaginal discharge.

2. **Vaginal spotting or bleeding.**

3. **Constant, dull lower back pain.**

4. **Pelvic or lower abdominal pressure.**

5. **Five or more contractions (sensations of her abdomen tightening) in an hour.**

6. **Her water breaks or she is leaking fluid.** This can happen in a gush or a trickle of fluid because the membrane around the babies breaks or tears. Here's a little something that we learned: urine smells, but amniotic fluid does not.

Again, remember that your role is to be able to speak up for your partner and her needs. When she might be hesitant to call or feels unsure about what she is experiencing, be the voice of reason and gently assure her that making a call to her doctor is always the best course of action.

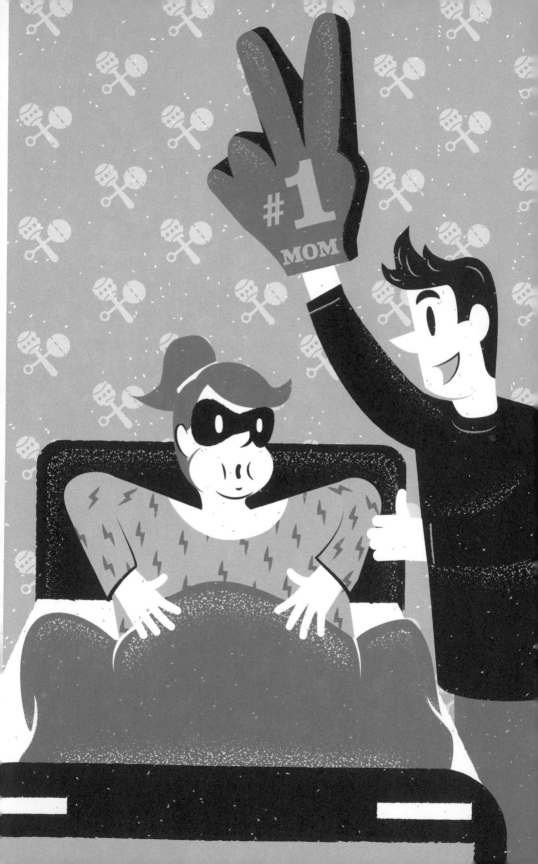

CHAPTER TWO
DELIVERY DAY!

It's game day. The warm-up is over. Those long months of preparation have come and gone. Now you are face-to-face with the reality that, in the very near future, you're going to be a dad of not one but two newborns. Delivery day is 100 percent about mom but that doesn't mean you won't be emotional too.

We both were excited and nervous right before our C-sections. Our husbands were stoically calm and focused the day of, being supportive and appearing relaxed through our deliveries. After the fact, however, they admitted they were really freaking out inside. Thoughts like, "Do I go with Baby A? Or do I wait until Baby B gets here? Can I touch my babies? What about my partner—how do I take care of all three at the same time?" flooded their minds. Preparedness gives you a sense of control and eases nerves when things get off track. Game-time decisions can be thought through ahead of time, helping you function calmly if something unexpected arises.

Throughout your partner's pregnancy you will want to be an active participant in doctor's appointments and have a thorough understanding of her needs and wants during labor and delivery. Advocacy is your new middle name. Prepare yourself now to speak up for her wishes and help her have the delivery experience that she wants.

This entire chapter is dedicated to preparing you for the big day. Start talking to other families, men and women alike, so that you can have a full understanding of labor and delivery, especially if you have friends that birthed multiples. No two experiences are the same. The important thing here is to take each person's account for what it's worth while keeping your expectations realistic. What happened to them won't necessarily happen to you.

When the day comes, everyone's focus will be on the mom and babies. You'll have plenty to do at the hospital, be it assisting in tandem feedings, making trips to the NICU while your partner sleeps, or keeping the text chain up-to-date. Shortly after birth, your life will return to a relatively normal state, while mom has to endure hormonal shifts and live with two babies attached to her nipples. Things come full circle and the extra effort put forward during labor, delivery, and postpartum healing helps everyone in the long run.

Dad's Role During Labor

More than coaching her through the "hee, hee, hoooos," your job is to be the team manager. Moral support, encouragement, and extra love are what she needs most. Your role is to remain calm and collected even if you are secretly freaking out.

If you took some time to prepare, the details of her birth plan should be fresh in your mind. Know the specifics about things like allergies to medication, pain management preferences, who she wants in the room, and what procedures (like antibiotic eye ointment, the vitamin K injection, circumcision) you may want performed after your babies are born. Take notes on your phone to help you remember when your mind goes to mush the minute you see your babies.

As you are refilling her ice chips, remember to do things like time contractions, take photos or videos, and keep your loved ones up-to-date via group texts. Keep her calm and comfortable, and spend your energy on things she needs to keep her focused on bringing two babies into the world.

Once Baby A arrives, you will probably have this urge to be with your newborn baby. However, with another one still on the way, don't be surprised if you feel overwhelmingly torn. This struggle will resonate throughout your life as a twin dad. The most useful advice we can give you is to go with your gut and do your best.

Meghan: Initially, I didn't want a video recording of our birth. At the last minute I pulled an audible. On the morning of, my husband threw our GoPro on his chest and captured amazing raw footage of our delivery. I put my editing skills to use and now we have a 10-minute video of that day. Our entire family loves to watch and yes, I still cry every single time.

What to Expect in the OR

It is not uncommon for twin births, even planned vaginal births, to take place in an operating room as a precaution. While your plans may not change, in 4 percent of twin births, one is delivered vaginally while the second one is delivered via Caesarean. Things change quickly, especially when delivering two babies, which is why doctors like to be as prepared as possible. Let's give you a rundown of what you will be doing and who may be in the OR for your twins' birth.

Before you ever step foot in the OR, you'll suit up: scrubs, a hairnet, and shoe covers. If your partner is having a C-section the hospital staff may get her settled and perform the spinal tap while you get dressed and ready. If you are planning a drug-free vaginal birth, be warned: some hospitals require an epidural be placed, without medication, in case things take a turn during labor or delivery.

Try not to be intimidated by the amount of medical staff making preparations when you walk in, but take comfort, as they all serve a specific purpose. It's quite a show.

You've got all the key players, including your OB, with possibly a supporting doc or medical student. In addition, you'll also have a handful of nurses in the room—something like one to two labor and delivery nurses and a pediatric nurse for each of your babies. An anesthesiologist will be present, as well as a nurse anesthetist to help with pain management or to prepare your partner if a C-section becomes necessary. Lastly, don't be surprised if additional medical students, pediatricians, and other specialists are in your OR, especially if your hospital doesn't have a NICU.

Dad's Hospital Bag

While your partner is busy focusing on having bags ready for herself and the babies, don't forget about you. Dad's comfort matters too. Think of your hospital stay like your annual guys' camping trip—exciting at first, then more and more uncomfortable as the trip goes on. Here's a list of all you might need to help make the hospital your home away from home.

★ **Bath towel.** You won't regret bringing one from home.

★ **Cameras.** Capturing new memories is part of your job!

★ **Chargers.** All the photo and video sharing will drain batteries fast. Invest in some extra-long cords too.

★ **Clothes.** You'll want a few changes of clothes in case your new babies do what babies do. Don't forget socks and underwear!

* **Deodorant.** Never a bad idea.

* **Entertainment.** Bring tablets, laptops, portable speaker, and/or books (like this one!).

* **Eye mask.** Medical staff come into your room at all hours throughout the night. You'll want to block out those fluorescent lights as much as you can.

* **Headphones with microphone.** For music and movies, plus hands-free talking.

* **Notepad and pen.** You never know when you might need to jot some stuff down.

* **Pajamas.** Privacy is scarce; you won't want to sleep in your skivvies.

* **Pillow.** You may stay an extra night or two so you'll want to be comfortable.

* **Shower shoes or slippers.** Hospitals are like the gym and no one likes to walk around with bare feet.

* **Sleeping bag or sheets and blankets.** The pull-out cot and scratchy hospital sheets aren't very welcoming.

* **Snacks.** Depending on the hospital, food choices might be slim.

* **Tennis ball.** Roll out tight spots in your back after spending several days on the pull-out cot.

* **Tennis shoes.** For the operating room.

* **Toiletries.** Bring shampoo, conditioner, body wash, toothbrush, toothpaste, floss, face wash, etc.

Managing a NICU Stay

Back in chapter 1, we talked about finding the perfect hospital, emphasizing the importance of having a NICU. We hope you have found something suitable. We cannot predict whether you will be faced with this challenge, nor can we predict the duration of your stay, but we can tell you that it will be an incredibly trying time for both of you.

Up until this point, your relationship has withstood the test of a twin pregnancy, maybe even infertility, and many other of life's challenges. This NICU stay is no different. It's crucial that you have the strength to advocate for yourself, for your partner, and for your babies.

On the other side of the coin, however, is having the self-awareness to know your own limitations. Through your partner's pregnancy and during delivery, you have been the foundation that keeps the house from falling, yet you are only human. Now, rely on your village—that network of family, friends, or even a therapist who can help alleviate your stress until you bring your babies home.

Consider the following section your crash course in NICU care. This section tackles a lot: the medical jargon, common NICU complications you might expect, and the pertinent staff that will be a part of your babies' medical team. Our hope is that you won't need much in this section. But, should you experience the NICU, we hope this information helps you navigate that experience.

NICU TIPS

Every twin parent wants to welcome healthy newborns into the world. That is the goal for your medical team too. However, sometimes life has different plans and babies are born a bit early or needing specialized medical care. Learning that your babies will require NICU care can feel overwhelming and anxiety producing. It's an emotional rollercoaster. We've gathered the following advice from parents who have been there:

★ Take an active role in your babies' medical care by attending rounds daily.

★ Use the nurses, an impartial authority, to act as a buffer for overbearing family members when you don't have the energy to tell people they cannot visit.

★ Make friends with the charge nurses and use them to navigate challenging situations with staff.

★ Learn the specific rules of your particular NICU. When can you be there? Who is allowed to visit you? What can you bring for your babies (clothes, blankets, etc.)?

★ Immediately ask how and when you can take on a role in caring for your babies (feeding, changing, etc.).

★ Use group texts to communicate updates to important family and friends.

★ Seek out support from friends or loved ones who've been there before or find support groups online. The r/NICUparents group on Reddit.com is a fantastic resource.

★ Save your FMLA paperwork for your pediatrician. Getting this paperwork signed probably won't happen in the NICU.

★ Ask questions and take notes. While you won't be sent home to fend for yourself without support, your baby's time in the NICU is your time to learn.

★ Your babies will be on a strict schedule, so get familiar with it. This will help you maintain your baby's schedule at home.

★ As you are preparing to go home, if you can, ask to room-in with your babies to get used to caring for your newborns with medical professionals nearby.

★ Prepare for going home by choosing health care providers ahead of time and gathering and getting to know all the necessary equipment and medications your babies will need.

★ Have a discussion as a couple (before going home) about who you want around on discharge day and the days following.

★ If one twin is leaving and one is staying, try to create a schedule so that you as a dad feel that you are making time and meeting the needs of both of your babies.

Important NICU Terminology

While there will be a large number of people involved in your babies' care for the foreseeable future, you and your partner are the most integral part of their medical team. Being informed and involved is your best defense. Medical jargon will be thrown around all day long and having a basic understanding of these terms will make you a better advocate. VerywellFamily.com provides some of the most common terms you'll hear and their definitions.

★ **A's and B's.** This is a slang term used by NICU nurses that refers to episodes of slower breathing and slower heart rates (apnea and bradycardia).

★ **Anemia.** Just like the condition in pregnancy, anemia refers to a low red blood cell count. Red blood cells are in charge of carrying oxygen to tissue.

★ **Apnea.** Apnea is a prolonged pause in breathing lasting more than 20 seconds. Premature infants commonly struggle with apnea, requiring monitoring and medication when appropriate.

★ **Aspirate.** This refers to a baby inhaling a foreign substance (milk or amniotic fluid) into their lungs.

★ **Bagging.** Bagging is done when a baby temporarily needs help breathing. Nurses pump air into the baby's lungs using oxygen and a rubber bag.

★ **Broviac (central catheter).** This is a thin tube placed in the upper chest used to administer or remove fluids from the body.

★ **Bilirubin.** Bilirubin is a waste product (yellowish in color) that forms when the body eliminates old red blood cells. Babies are placed under fluorescent lights (phototherapy) or on a biliblanket to reduce their bilirubin levels.

★ **Bradycardia.** Bradycardia is the slowing of a baby's heart rate.

★ **Corrected age.** Sometimes referred to as adjusted age, this is a baby's age according to gestation.

★ **CPAP (continuous positive airway pressure).** A CPAP is a ventilator that helps your baby's lungs expand properly. It does not actually breathe for the baby.

★ **Cyanosis.** Cyanosis is a blue tone in the skin that results from a drop in oxygen levels.

★ **Echocardiogram.** This is a test performed using sound waves to look at your baby's heart through the chest wall. It is performed similarly to an ultrasound.

★ **ETT (endotracheal tube).** This is a tube that goes into a baby's mouth or nose to get oxygen into the lungs.

★ **Extubate.** Extubating is the removal of a tube that went through the baby's mouth or nose into the trachea.

★ **Gavage feedings.** Feedings that provide nutrition through a tube passed through the baby's nose or mouth into their stomach.

★ **Guthrie test/neonatal.** The Guthrie test is a newborn screening test performed by pricking the baby's heel to draw blood in order to detect a variety of congenital diseases.

★ **Hypotension.** Low blood pressure.

★ **Intubate.** Intubating refers to the insertion of a tube into the trachea through the baby's nose or mouth to help air reach the lungs.

★ **Isolette or incubator.** This is an enclosed "bed" that helps a premature baby maintain body temperature.

★ **I's and O's.** This is more NICU slang that refers to the amount of liquid that a baby takes in compared to the amount they pee or poop.

★ **Kangaroo care.** Kangaroo care, otherwise known as skin-to-skin, is where a baby is placed on the bare skin of their mother or father.

★ **NPO.** NPO is an acronym for *nil per os* or "nothing by mouth." If a baby is marked NPO, all nutrition will be given intravenously.

★ **PICC line (peripherally inserted central catheter).** A PICC line is used when antibiotics, IV therapy, or nutrition are administered for a long time. It is inserted through a vein and eventually advanced through larger veins toward the heart.

★ **Pulse oximetry.** Pulse oximetry is a noninvasive way to monitor your babies' oxygen saturation.

★ **Perinatal.** This term refers to the weeks before and after birth.

★ **PKU (phenylketonuria).** PKU is a rare disorder where babies cannot tolerate one of the amino acids, leading to elevated levels in their blood. A routine blood test using special paper, usually performed 24 to 72 hours after birth, is used to test for this condition. This test is usually repeated for premature babies around two weeks and again at four weeks of age.

★ **Premature/preterm/preemie.** This refers to a baby born before 37 weeks gestation.

★ **"Priming the gut."** This is more slang terminology referring to slowly starting feedings for a baby in order to prepare their digestive system to fully function.

★ **Reflux.** Spitting up is common in premature infants as a result of a backflow of the baby's stomach contents.

★ **Suctioning.** Suctioning involves removing secretions from your baby's mouth, nose, or lungs with a bulb syringe or a suctioning catheter.

★ **Surfactants.** Surfactants are lubricants in the lungs. Respiratory distress syndrome (RDS) is a common breathing complication in premature babies due to a lack of surfactants in their lungs.

★ **TPN (total parenteral nutrition).** TPN is given when a baby should not receive feedings and fluid by mouth. This method of feeding bypasses the gastrointestinal tract.

★ **Ventilator.** A ventilator is a machine that helps a baby breathe by pumping oxygen into the lungs through a tube.

★ **Wean.** In the NICU, weaning refers to the process of removing a baby from a ventilator and incubator.

The NICU Medical Team

Your babies will have a stacked team of medical professionals. It's not likely that you will interact with each and every team member treating your babies on a daily basis, but at some level, each of these professionals is closely monitoring their progress.

★ **Nurse.** Your baby's nurse will be a specially trained registered nurse (RN) who is in charge of delivering nursing care to your infants. They typically work 12-hour shifts.

★ **Clinical nurse IV.** Also referred to as a charge nurse, this person oversees the care of each baby. They are available to assist nurses and doctors as well as help parents problem solve.

★ **Clinical nurse specialist.** This is a nurse with an advanced degree in infant nursing care. They manage care in special clinical situations.

★ **Discharge coordinator.** This nurse plans for discharge with the family and medical team. Their primary job is to make sure everyone is ready to go home.

★ **Nursing care technician (NCT).** This person is the unit's secretary.

★ **Nurse manager.** This nurse is in charge of supervising the unit's staff, setting schedules, managing patient care, and making management decisions.

★ **Consulting physician (cardiologist, neurologist, ophthalmologist, etc.).** A consulting physician would be a doctor trained in a discipline other than pediatrics.

★ **Neonatologist.** This is a pediatrician who cares for premature and sick babies.

★ **Pediatrician.** A pediatrician is a doctor who manages the health care of children.

★ **Social worker.** A social worker is a clinician with a master's degree in social work who helps the families emotionally manage their situation. This person can also help with community resources and finances.

★ **Case manager.** A case manager helps deal with insurance as well as discharge and home care.

★ **Parent liaison.** The parent liaison is a NICU staff member who has had their own infant require NICU care.

Common NICU Disorders

These are some likely reasons a baby might end up in the NICU. We encourage you to discuss your concerns with the medical professionals in charge of your baby's medical health care. Whatever you do, don't be that guy and Google everything; you'll only freak yourself out. When in doubt just go ask a nurse or a doctor.

★ **Apnea.** Irregular breathing patterns are common in premature babies.

★ **Congenital defects.** Physical defects present at birth.

★ **Congenital heart disease.** Babies born with a defect in the form of heart function.

★ **Intraventricular hemorrhage (IVH).** Bleeding in the normal hollow spaces of the brain. The most common hemorrhages are minor, causing little to no harm.

★ **Jaundice.** A condition where bilirubin (a waste product caused when the body eliminates old red blood cells) enters the blood.

★ **Meconium aspiration.** At times, while still in utero, babies may poop (otherwise known as meconium). If this substance is aspirated into a baby's lungs, it can cause breathing difficulties. Suction, by placing a tube into the baby's lungs, may be required to treat this condition.

★ **Necrotizing enterocolitis (NEC).** This is an infection in the wall of the intestines that can spread into a baby's blood.

★ **Patent ductus arteriosus.** Before birth, oxygen is supplied by mom through the placenta. Blood is moved away from the lungs into the rest of the body via a vessel called the ductus arteriosus, which normally closes shortly after birth. In premature babies, this vessel can fail to close.

★ **Pneumothorax.** This is otherwise referred to as an "air leak" into the space between the baby's lungs and chest wall. If the space is large enough, air may need to be removed with a tube or needle placed into the chest.

★ **Respiratory distress syndrome (RDS).** This is the most common medical complication in premature babies and refers to a lack of surfactant (lubricant) in a baby's lungs.

★ **Retinopathy of prematurity (ROP).** This is a problem of the retina (the back part of the eye that "sees") that occurs in premature infants. At times surgery may be necessary, but most babies who are born with it get better over time.

Stay Positive

Randy Pausch, the late motivational author and professor at Carnegie Mellon University, put it perfectly: "We cannot change the cards we are dealt, just how we play the hand." We wish we could wave a magic wand that would guarantee perfect outcomes for you and your newborn babies, but that simply isn't realistic. Even in the toughest moments, positive vibes will be your guiding light. Easier said than done, we know. This time away from your newborns will likely test you and your partner to the core, but it's important to remain positive, not only for yourself but for your relationship.

Finding a way to look at your NICU stay with some positivity can really change your experience and boost your emotional stamina. As a couple, turn your focus onto the small wins; every little milestone that your babies meet is monumentally important. Celebrating those along the way will change your perspective and reduce your stress. Did your babies gain weight today? Did they sleep through the night without pulling out a tube? NICU milestones, as small as they may seem, are significant. Focusing on these little silver linings has a way of changing your worrisome thoughts into hopeful ones.

Remember, this is the very best place your babies can be when they need specialized medical care. Yes, the machines may look and sound intimidating. However, if you try to see the technology and teams of doctors as tools to help your babies go home healthy, you will feel more comfortable having your babies in the NICU. As long as you are willing to adapt, you will be ready for anything that is thrown your way. No matter what, know that these babies are super lucky because you are their dad.

Postpartum Depression

Your partner's hormones will shift post-delivery, which can lead to intense emotional swings. In fact, postpartum mood disorders like the "baby blues," postpartum depression, and anxiety are common complications of childbirth. The Mayo Clinic states that mothers of multiples are more susceptible to facing postpartum depression or anxiety and have 43 percent greater odds of having moderate to severe postpartum mood disorders.

Baby blues, typically showing up within the first two or three days after delivery, often manifest in mood swings, unexplained crying, anxiety, or sleeping difficulties. The symptoms typically last for a few weeks.

Postpartum depression, often initially mistaken for the baby blues, is characterized by more intense, longer-lasting symptoms. These symptoms can show up during pregnancy, within a few days or weeks, but can manifest as late as a year after birth. They begin to interfere with a mother's ability to care for her babies and handle daily tasks. Symptoms include:

★ Severe mood swings and/or a depressed mood

★ Excessive crying

★ Difficulty bonding with the new babies

★ Extreme fluctuations in appetite (either loss of appetite or excessive eating)

★ Sleeping difficulties (insomnia or excessive sleeping)

★ Feelings of hopelessness

★ Anxiety or panic attacks

★ Trouble concentrating

* Intense irritability

* Thoughts of suicide

New moms, especially those learning to care for two babies or having babies requiring NICU care, may struggle to recognize that what they are experiencing is symptomatic of postpartum depression. Waiting and hoping things will improve isn't the best course of action. Again, your role as the supportive partner and new dad is to be an advocate, especially when your partner can't advocate for herself. You see this person daily. If something seems off, start talking to medical professionals about solutions.

Men are able to develop postpartum depression as well. According to PostpartumDepression.org, around 25 percent of men develop postpartum depression, but only about 10 percent of cases are actually recorded. You don't have to go through this alone and remain quiet about it. We mention paternal postpartum depression (PPPD) or paternal postnatal depression (PPND) not to scare you but for awareness. Take it seriously and get help when you need it. If you're not sure who to ask, start with a nurse. Many hospitals have trained staff on call to counsel patients at times like this. Your mental health is incredibly important.

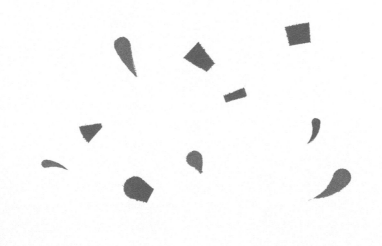

They're Home!
Your First Night as a Twin Dad

One of the greatest things a dad can experience is bringing home his newborn twins from the hospital. Carrying two occupied car seats over the threshold suddenly makes everything feel complete. Plan for this moment by having discussions as a couple before that day arrives. Consider what you might need, what might feel overwhelming to you, and what might be comforting as you begin to settle in as a family.

Do you want visitors right away or would you prefer to wait a few days? Exhaustion has already taken its toll a little, so inviting others into your home might not be ideal. On the flip side, having visitors who are helpful might give you a minute to catch your breath, nap, and shower.

Will it be helpful to have out-of-town guests staying with you? Just be sure to set clear boundaries with family and friends. While they are there to be helpful, overbearing relatives can easily take over. Take the reins because you won't get these moments back. You and your partner will want to own all of the "firsts."

Prepare freezer meals or ask a loved one to have your fridge fully stocked prior to your arrival at home so that you have the energy you will need to take care of your newborn babies and your healing partner.

Whether you decide to sleep with the babies in your bedroom or you want them in the nursery from the get-go, you will be up quite a few times. It gets easier, but at first you may obsessively check to be sure they are breathing. There is nothing better than watching your new babies sleep in your home that first night.

Adjusting to your new life is going to take time. While you and your partner find your groove, keep your expectations realistic. Set the bar where you can expect to have beautiful moments met by messiness and chaos. Sleep deprivation and self-doubt can make the novelty wear off fast. There will be moments when you both roll up your sleeves and go all in, and moments when your individual strengths will need to shine. The key to keeping your partnership intact is to stick together, lean on each other, and give each other a break from time to time.

Meghan: *Heading home from the hospital with our newborn twins was an exciting and nerve-racking experience. All of a sudden we were responsible for keeping two babies safe, and driving with them? Well, that was a whole new ball game. We realized that we had a lot to learn. The discharge nurse warned us that babies can get sunburned in the car. Having not known or even considered that, our focused turned to keeping the sun off our newborns. My husband drove a whopping 25 miles per hour, stopping along the way to adjust our makeshift sunshades. When we arrived home, we discovered that one of our babies wasn't even buckled into his car seat! There we were, two new, exhausted twin parents who checked six times that Baby A was buckled safely but, distracted by the damn sunshades, failed to double-check Baby B's buckle. Things like this happen. The best we can do is learn from our mistakes and move on.*

Jenn: *On the day that we went home from the hospital with our twins, my parents called to check in on us. Because they lived close by, they offered to bring by groceries, diapers, and any other essentials we may have missed. Our first instinct was to graciously ask that they wait a day or two, but after we thought about it for a moment, the thought of a long, hot shower and time for a nap in our own bed won out! Once home, we realized that we didn't plan all that well. Our fridge was empty and all of the newborn clothes (naively we believed [the twins] would not be small enough for preemie sizes) weren't going to work. Within an hour my parents walked in with groceries and Babies "R" Us bags. The greatest gift they gave us was the opportunity to get ourselves back to neutral before we tackled parenthood with two all by ourselves.*

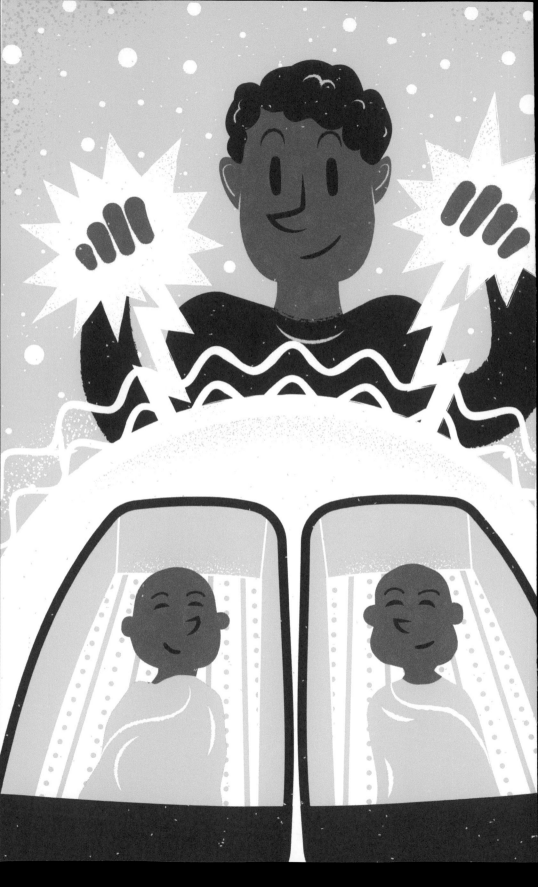

CHAPTER THREE

NOW WHAT?

Do you hear that? It's the roar of our congratulatory applause because, well, it's official! You are now a *twin dad*. After the dust settles and you come off that amazing post-birth high, roll up those sleeves because the real work starts now. Parents of twins need to know that an all-hands-on-deck approach is necessary while you adjust to parenthood and begin to define your individual roles. New parents have big shoes to fill, but you especially, as dad, will do some heavy lifting while everyone settles in. We designed this chapter to help you do that by covering dad-specific issues you'll face in the first few weeks. So, if you are worried that you'll have trouble bonding with your babies right away or that you'll get your twins mixed up, the following pages will help you navigate your new role. Take a deep breath, soak up these first moments of fatherhood, and get ready for a wild ride.

Bonding with Babies

Dad's most important job after birth, aside from caring for mom while she heals, is to begin bonding with their babies, as a pair and individually. Moms get a nine-month head start in the intimate connection department, so dad has to make an effort to develop a relationship with his babies. Bonding helps with babies' physical, emotional, and mental development while simultaneously reducing a parent's stress and increasing their confidence.

When we work with new parents, we often hear anxiety and worry that dads won't feel a strong attachment right way. This is a perfectly normal way to feel. Everyone bonds at their own pace. Many dads instinctively jump in there, while other dads aren't sure where to begin. If things don't click right away, relax. You're a dad now. Here are some tips to help you get connected.

★ **Skin-to-skin contact.** Placing your naked baby on your bare chest is a multisensory experience for babies. Holding one or both of your babies releases hormones—oxytocin, prolactin, and endorphins—that help develop bonds.

★ **Singing to babies.** Your voice soothes your babies, who recognize it from their time in the womb. Tune up those pipes and sing your favorite hits while holding your babies close and looking into their eyes.

★ **Gentle playtime.** Newborns enjoy short periods of play. Talking during tummy time, giving them a tour of the house, and making silly faces are all ways to engage with a newborn.

★ **Reading to babies.** Research shows that literacy development can never start too early. Break out your childhood favorites and spend time reading aloud. Reading is a good step to add to bedtime routines.

★ **Mirror movements and facial expression.** The first step in developing communication with your newborns is mirroring their movements, facial expressions, and cooing sounds.

How to Tell Identical Twins Apart

Having identical twins takes invasive baby questioning to a whole new level. You'll constantly hear "Are they twins?" followed by "Are they identical?" and "How can you tell?" In no time at all, you'll develop an arsenal of sarcastic answers to these questions. The truth is all new twin dads, at some level, worry about this. Fortunately, if you aren't able to tell them apart right away, you'll figure it out shortly thereafter.

The majority of our clients with identical twins, both moms and dads alike, simply know who is who. It is instinct. It is unlikely you'll have to paint toenails or tattoo their heels with permanent marker to tell your twins apart.

From the beginning, the hospital staff will keep them organized and labeled. Hospital bracelets and the nursing staff's typical routine of keeping Baby A on the left and Baby B on the right helps parents out immensely. Once you have settled into your room, look for small birthmarks and distinct physical features. After a short period, even with sleep deprivation setting in, your twins will become easily distinguishable. Their cries, coos, and eating and sleeping schedules will be your indicators, telling you who is who without a second thought.

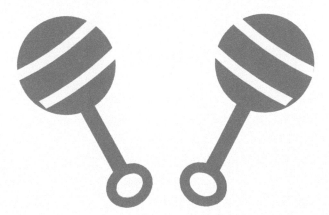

Put the Work in Paperwork

Your new role as Chief Dad in Charge isn't all snuggles and cuddles. Children come with a hefty price tag and soon mountains of paperwork will start pouring in. Here you are with two new babies and a partner who is recovering from the birth, and now you have to find a way to tackle the expenses. Feeling overwhelmed is natural.

We highly recommend that you temporarily take on the role of family CFO, even if you and your partner have equally divided the burden of your household bills. After giving birth to two babies, your partner will be going through an insurmountable adjustment as she deals with feeding (or breastfeeding), healing, and hormones. You tracking and paying bills, even temporarily, will be an immense relief to your partner.

Get organized. Learn how to make spreadsheets for bill and budget tracking and invest in accordion folders or file boxes for your paperwork. As your mailbox fills up, immediately label and file things away, then track what you've received and what you've paid on a spreadsheet.

Your system can be simple or something like your CPA might use, but either way having a system is essential. Growing your family exponentially can shift your budget quite a bit. Diapers, formula, medical bills, and child care will quickly drain your finances. You'll sleep better at night knowing where your money goes. And, at this point in the game, sleep is something you can't afford to lose.

Paternity Leave 101

Paternity leave is a highly coveted benefit that varies from job to job. You might find yourself staring at a few weeks off with your newborn twins depending on where you live and work. Early on in the pregnancy, do some research. Find out how much time you are allotted, if any. Is it paid or unpaid? Can you take time off sporadically, over the course of a year, or do you need to take all of your time at once? Your specific circumstances, like the twins requiring NICU time or your part-ner going back to work soon, may drive how that time is used.

Speaking from experience, bringing two babies home at the same time works best with an all-hands-on-deck approach to help in those first few weeks. Regardless of what flexibility you have with your leave, you'll want to use some of that time when your family first comes home. You'll be essential in caring for your babies while your partner heals and everyone adjusts to your new life.

Some dads choose to use all of their time in the beginning while others take some time initially and then more later on when sleep challenges arise or to take trips to visit family. A word to the wise: don't let societal norms make you feel like you *shouldn't* use all of your time away from work. If you have it, use it. Work will always be there.

Nannies, Grannies, or Day Care?

Nannies, grannies, and day care, oh my! Most families need to think about child care options for when mom goes back to work. For fami-lies with multiples, it is even more complex due to the added expense and challenges that come along with having two babies requiring care. Finding the option that best fits your family takes time and research. Don't let this decision linger until the last minute; discuss it early and often.

Child care options can vary; each option has its pros and cons as well as an associated cost (emotional and financial) to consider before deciding for your family.

★ **Family helpers.** Family members may offer child care for a minimal cost or even for free, making this a desirable and cost-effective choice. This gives parents a sense of security, knowing that their babies are cared for by someone they know and love. On the flip side, consider how trusted family (say, your mother-in-law) will uphold your wishes during the day. Conversations can get sticky when a well-intentioned grandparent wants to show off your babies while you need them home napping on a schedule. If you choose this route, have explicit instructions and be direct. Be sure to offer an "out" for your loved one should they burn out. The last thing you want is a strained relationship because your parenting styles differ.

★ **In-home nanny.** Finding in-home child care has wonderful benefits. It can ease your anxiety about schedules, make drop-off/pick-up convenient, and help minimize illness. On the downside, a nanny can be costly, especially someone with experience for two babies. Paying nannies is a more complicated venture, requiring families to think through the tax implications of having an employee of your family. Consider what might happen when your nanny gets sick, wants to take a vacation, or quits without notice. While these scenarios aren't ideal, they happen and you need to be prepared.

★ **Nanny shares.** Families can join efforts to hire one nanny for all of their children and share the cost. Nanny shares allow your babies to socialize with other children but they can be complicated. You will need to explicitly work out details like whose home the children will be in (or if that location should alternate), how the other children's schedule will affect your established routine, or what to do if someone in the nanny share gets sick.

★ **Traditional (center-based) day care.** Day care centers, typically the most expensive option, can vary depending on their ownership and affiliation. Aside from accreditation, look for centers that meet the AAP infant-to-caregiver ratio recommendation, allow parents to drop by unannounced, have clear discipline and illness policies, and have a staff that is certified in early childhood development and CPR. Some day care centers offer a sibling discount (often 10 percent). Keep in mind that you are paying for your spot in a traditional center, meaning that you will typically pay for days your children are not present.

The Pet-Friendly Introduction

Your fur babies were once the center of your universe and that is about to change dramatically. Becoming human parents doesn't mean that they have to suffer. It's important that you prepare *everything* and *everyone* in your home for a new lifestyle. In the weeks leading up to your anticipated due date, set your pets up for success. Give them the time and attention they deserve to be ready for this major adjustment.

★ Let your pets be a part of the pregnancy by allowing them to sniff and snuggle with the bump.

★ Allow your pets time to become comfortable in the nursery, even before your babies are born. Consider adding a pet bed in the nursery and spend time acclimating your dog or cat to their safe place within the new room.

★ Give your pets their own space somewhere (baby-free) in your home. A dog bed in your room; a kennel in the living room. Give your pet somewhere to go and be alone that is only theirs.

★ Before your babies are discharged, bring home used hospital blankets for your pets to snuggle with, to introduce the new smells.

★ When you bring your babies home, go inside to greet your pet without the babies at first. Then plan a *short* meet and greet for your pets. Let your animals get used to the new sounds your babies will make.

★ Allow an adjustment period. Your pets don't need to instantly accept or be comfortable with your babies.

CONTINUED >>

★ Keep your pet's rules and expectations the same once your babies are home. Don't banish them to the backyard or a kennel for countless hours a day. Allow them to roam around your home—supervised, but as normal.

★ Maintain your pet's routine. If morning walks are part of your daily ritual, do your best to keep those intact. It'll be good for the babies too.

★ Give your pets attention *away* from your babies.

★ Be sure you never leave your pets (as trusted as they may be) unsupervised with your infants.

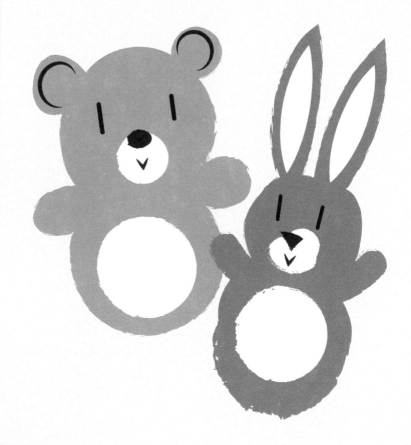

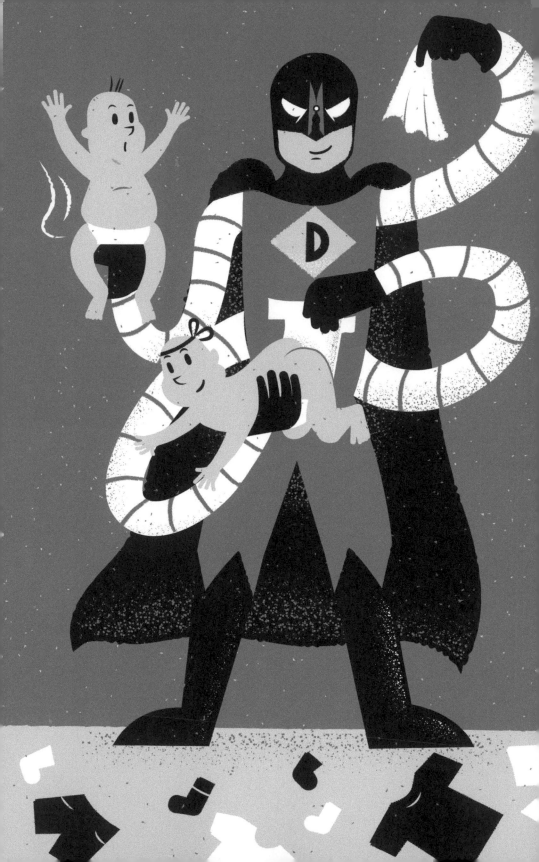

CHAPTER FOUR
ZERO TO THREE MONTHS

One day you'll only remember the meaningful firsts of being a new twin dad and not the exhaustion or the millions of diapers. The first few months of fatherhood are a blur of sleeping and feeding schedules, tracking who pooped when, and figuring out how to fall asleep to the whine of a breast pump.

Don't get us wrong, these early months are unforgettable. There will be moments of major success. Parenting is a wacky science experiment based on trial and error, so again, knowledge is power. The better prepared you are now, the better off you will be. There will be a lot of beautiful, amazing firsts and plenty of frustrated learning experiences in the coming months as you start to figure out how to "dad."

Milestones

The following milestones are established by the CDC. These guidelines help parents track growth and development but always remember *babies develop at their own pace.* And yes, with two developing side by side, it is easy to make comparisons and get freaked out. Hit the pause button for a moment to remember that your twins are two individuals who are developing differently and will do so their entire lives.

SOCIAL AND EMOTIONAL

To your newborn babies, the world is a large, unknown place. Your babies are relying on you to show them that you are the person who cares for them and meets their needs. This trust is crucial to their social and emotional development. At zero to three months your babies will begin to smile socially, and they'll feel comforted by, and enjoy playing with, familiar adults. Babies learn to express themselves by imitating your facial expressions and movements. They may even begin to coo and repeat vowel sounds when you talk or play. Eat these moments up because they go by fast.

VISUAL AND HEARING

Believe it or not, your babies will start to communicate immediately. Each day they will slowly start to put the pieces together with sights and sounds. They'll begin listening and responding to voices, smiling or turning toward you when they hear your voice. Around one month, your twins will probably like to look at bold black-and-white patterns. By two months, their eyes will become more coordinated and they will start to track objects as they use their hands.

MOVEMENT AND PHYSICAL DEVELOPMENT

Babies will begin to open and shut their hands and respond positively (see: smiling) to touch. They will start to grasp objects or even hold a toy for a few moments. Your babies will begin to hold their heads up when laying on their tummies, kick and stretch their legs, and start to bring their hands to their mouths.

Meghan: Those first few months with the boys [were] when our teamwork really began. We thought we were a strong team through years of infertility, but soon realized our bonding got rock-solid when we became twin parents. After late-night feedings and diaper changes, we caught ourselves high-fiving each other in the dark hallway celebrating that we nailed yet another night waking! Matt would help the boys latch, then we'd each take a baby and supplement with formula, diaper change, and head back to bed! Small victories at 3:00 a.m. were big wins in our new parenting roles. Our bond as a couple got stronger by the day.

Doctor, Doctor

Just when you thought the countless visits to the doctor during your partner's pregnancy had come to an end, you brought home two babies. The American Academy of Pediatrics recommends that newborns are seen 3 to 5 days after birth and then regularly at 1, 2, 4, 6, 9, 12, 15, 18, and 24 months. During each of these checkups you can expect the pediatrician to:

★ **Take measurements.** The doctors will measure length (equal to the baby's height), weight, and head circumference. These statistics will be tracked against infants of the same age to rule out problems with growth.

★ **Assess development.** You will be asked questions based on your child's age to help the doctor gauge development. Discuss concerns about missed or delayed milestones during these appointments.

★ **Assess behavior.** The doctors will observe and discuss your babies' behavior to rule out psychological or behavioral concerns.

★ **Physical exam.** A thorough head-to-toe physical exam will be given. The doctors will look at your babies' eyes, ears, mouth, skin, heart, lungs, belly, hips, and legs. They will also check the soft spot on your babies' heads until the skull fuses together around 12 months.

★ **One-month-visit vaccines.** The babies will get a tuberculosis (TB) test and the second dose of the hepatitis B (hep B) vaccine, the first of which they received at birth. The TB test requires the doctor to inject an inactive strain of TB into your baby's arm.

★ **Two-month-visit vaccines.** Okay, Dad, get ready. This appointment comes with a hefty dose of important immunizations. While babies generally tolerate all of the shots without significant side effects, be prepared for a fussier baby (or two) who will need lots of cuddles and maybe a dose of Tylenol. At the two-month visit, your babies will get the first dose of rotavirus (RV) vaccine, diphtheria, tetanus toxoids, acellular pertussis vaccine (DTaP), haemophilus influenzae type b conjugate vaccine (Hib), pneumococcal vaccine (PCV), and inactivated poliovirus vaccine (IPV). While it seems like a large number of needles, many of these can be combined into fewer shots. As always, chat with your doctor about any questions or concerns regarding the vaccination schedule.

Sleeping

With twins, well, you'll join Team No Sleep a bit sooner than most new parents. Babies aren't born knowing how to be champion sleepers, they are taught. What you teach in those first few months can help set your babies up for success down the road when it's time for sleep training. Consider this Infant Sleep 101 so you know what to expect from your newborn twins.

What If Milestones Are Missed?

As a twin dad, you'll have a front row seat to watch two babies develop. Talk with your doctor during all of those newborn appointments and ask any and all questions. As a parent of multiples, you're in a unique position. Comparisons fool you into thinking there are problems, when in reality everything may be perfectly normal. If there were fine print, it would tell you that babies grow and develop at different rates. Your twins (identical and fraternal alike) are no different.

Twin parents often find themselves comparing their babies because they are the same age. One might be just lifting their head while the other is starting to track you with their eyes and smiling at your voice. Remember, these are two completely unique humans who might not meet expected milestones at the same time. Prematurity, health issues at birth, and general genetic makeup all play a role in growth and development. Let professionals diagnose developmental delays, not Dr. Google. And if your babies do need help, doctors will be the ones who can help you figure out the best plan for your family.

Infant sleep cycles are different from adults'. According to the Sleep Foundation, they last around 45 to 60 minutes, unlike the cycles of adults, which are typically 70 to 100 minutes long. What makes infant sleep so challenging is getting the babies to sleep *and* keeping them asleep through those sleep cycles. This is especially challenging at night when babies spend 50 percent of their sleep in light, active sleep. Their sleep is fragmented and unpredictable as sleep cycles develop. After six to eight weeks you can expect things to settle down and begin developing a real schedule for your babies.

Yes, you will be powering through sleepless nights, but all hope is not lost either. It's amazing how well you can function on little sleep as a new parent. Spending some time understanding infant sleep now will help you tackle the monumental task of teaching your babies how to be good sleepers.

SUDDEN INFANT DEATH SYNDROME (SIDS)

It's natural for new parents to incessantly check on their sleeping newborns to see if they're breathing. Parents worry; it's part of the job. SIDS, or the sudden death of an infant, usually in their sleep, is a real phenomenon that keeps parents on edge. While there is no foolproof way to prevent SIDS, The Mayo Clinic suggests that the following simple precautions will reduce the risk of something happening to your babies.

★ Lay babies down to sleep on their backs.

★ Babies' beds should be firm, with a tight-fitting sheet. Leave extra bedding, blankets, and stuffed animals out of their sleeping space.

★ Consider allowing your baby to sleep with a pacifier.

★ Room-in or co-sleep with your babies in a baby lounger-type contraption until they are six months old. If you choose to co-sleep, be sure to discuss safe co-sleeping practices with your pediatrician and use co-sleepers.

★ Prevent your babies from overheating with appropriate pajamas and a room temperature ranging from 68 to 72 degrees Fahrenheit.

INFANT SLEEP CUES

Think wearing babies out helps them sleep better? Wrong. Overtiredness causes the body to produce more cortisol and adrenaline to stay awake, which exhausted parents most certainly don't want. When you see yawning or eye rubbing, or if your babies begin to avoid eye contact with you, begin to get your babies ready for sleep even if it's outside the "normal" schedule.

DROWSY BUT AWAKE

The saying "practice makes permanent" definitely applies when teaching new babies healthy sleep habits. It's never too early to use best sleep practices. Look for sleep cues. As soon as you see eye rubbing and yawns, move to a dark room, maybe swaddle your babies, feed and rock them until they are in a drowsy state (not asleep), then lay them down. This practice is fundamental in teaching your babies to fall asleep on their own instead of in your arms.

DAY VS. NIGHT CONFUSION

Spending close to nine months in a dark womb doesn't teach babies about the differences between daytime and nighttime. Internal clocks inherently tell our bodies when it is time to sleep and be awake within 24-hour intervals. Babies aren't born with a developed internal clock and will need help understanding the difference between day and night. During the day, keep the house bright, full of conversation, and activity. At night, when bedtime is nearing, turn down the lights and noise.

STARTLE REFLEX

Have you ever been startled awake by the feeling of falling? Babies are born with a startle (moro) reflex that can jolt them awake. Loud noises or the feeling of falling can cause babies to throw their arms and legs outward. Not to worry, this reflex generally disappears between three and six months, according to the Mayo Clinic. In the meantime, tightly swaddling your babies and putting them in a room filled with white noise can help.

BEDTIME ROUTINE

The earlier you introduce good sleep habits, the better. Babies thrive with routine. As early as two to three weeks, start implementing a soothing bedtime routine each time you lay your babies down to sleep.

Consistently using the same steps in the same order, like changing diapers, putting on pajamas (or sleep sacks, or swaddles), reading a story, and then wrapping things up with a feeding, helps signal to them that sleep is coming.

COLICKY BABIES AND SLEEP

Babies cry. There are no ifs, ands, or buts about it. However, the Mayo Clinic suggests that when a baby cries for more than three hours a day at least three days a week for three weeks, they likely have colic. If you have a colicky baby (or two) we advise that you do whatever you can to get them to sleep. Worry about getting routines back on track after the colic has passed.

Feeding

Now's the time to put those old bartending skills to good use. Whether you are feeding one baby or two with a bottle, breast, or a combination of both, your success lies in getting good information and professional support from the get-go. You need a basic understanding of your babies' nutritional needs and how they'll change within the first year.

HOW MUCH AND HOW OFTEN SHOULD BABIES EAT?

Have you ever left a sushi dinner feeling stuffed only to be starving an hour later? You can liken that experience to what your newborns are feeling. You will feed your babies around the clock, especially in the early days and weeks. Babies are born with stomachs the size of cherries, which grow to the size of a large egg by one month of age. The amount a baby needs to eat changes drastically in just the first month of life and will continue to change as the belly grows.

INFANT HUNGER CUES

Ever go to the grocery store on an empty stomach? Your missed hunger cues likely caused you to stroll the aisles and add extra snacks to your cart. Slightly hungry babies smack their lips together, opening their mouths to root or suck on anything nearby, whereas really hungry babies cry. The hungrier a baby gets, the fussier and more agitated they become. Like sleep, the earlier you recognize hunger cues and get babies fed, the easier things are for everyone.

BREASTFEEDING, FORMULA, OR BOTH

As a twin dad, you'll be needed at feeding time. The decision on how your twins will be fed (breastfeeding, formula, or both) is highly dependent on your partner, because your babies have to attach themselves to her nipples. Your role is to be helpful and supportive.

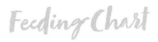

Feeding Chart

AGE	OUNCES IN A BOTTLE (APPROXIMATION)	NUMBER OF FEEDINGS PER DAY*	HOW OFTEN SHOULD BABIES EAT?	TOTAL OUNCES IN 24-HOUR PERIOD
0 to 2 days	1 to 3 ounces (30–60 mL)	8 to 12	1 to 3 hours	8 to 24 ounces
3 days to 4 weeks	2 to 3 ounces (60–90 mL)	8 to 10	2 to 4 hours	24 to 32 ounces
4 to 12 weeks	4 to 5 ounces (119–148 mL)	6 to 8	3 to 4 hours	24 to 32 ounces

Breastfed babies will need more frequent feedings per day.
Source: HerCottage.com

Bottle or breast, you are needed. You won't sit on the sidelines to watch the whole ordeal go down. With a breastfeeding mom, you will be useful in helping your partner learn to tandem breastfeed, squishing boobs into hamburgers to get babies to latch, positioning babies, or maybe reminding your partner which baby started on which breast at 1:00 a.m. You might have one champion breastfeeder and one that needs extra support. As much as possible, especially in the beginning, be a part of the conversations with a lactation consultant so that you are armed with information once you get home.

If you are exclusively formula feeding, or using formula as a supplement, you will become a pro at making and measuring bottles. You can help feed both babies or one at a time, help burp babies mid-feed, and get the bottles washed and ready for the next feed.

As you and your partner navigate the eat-sleep-poop routine, remember that you can be a voice of reason if things get stressful. Our husbands were unequivocally supportive of the choices we were making to feed our babies, but they also knew when to step in and offer support when our breastfeeding goals hit a snag.

Jenn: My breastfeeding journey was challenged from the beginning. After years of infertility, all I wanted was to have some control over how I fed our boys, so I set out to breastfeed for a year. Shortly into our journey, I struggled with low supply issues, and one of our babies lost weight. We were forced to supplement, but I didn't want to give up the fight either. I spent eight long months pumping six to eight times a day. Around the eight-month mark, after lots of tears on my end, my husband sat me down to have a supportive, yet frank conversation. Thanks to his honest, supportive, and empathetic tone, I was able to accept that I did the best I could. It was him saying that he was proud of what we had accomplished that put me at ease. Jordan had the wisdom to know that it was time to move on because it was taking a toll on me, emotionally, physically, and mentally.

FEEDING ON DEMAND VS. SCHEDULED FEEDINGS

There are two schools of thought when it comes to feeding babies, each having their benefits and challenges. While we are of the belief that scheduling is the secret to survival as a twin parent, adhering to a strictly scheduled approach can be challenging for breastfeeding moms, impacting their milk supply. On the flip side, however, twin moms who are feeding on demand can quickly become overwhelmed with having to constantly be available to feed two babies *all of the time.*

Feeding on demand, where you let your babies show you that they are hungry and eat until they are satisfied, is the best way to approach feedings in the early days, weeks, and months. This approach helps new mothers establish a full milk supply, ensures your babies are getting enough to eat, and encourages bonding. As your babies mature, around three to four months, more predictable patterns will begin to emerge, helping you set more of a schedule and routine. Be prepared for things to change frequently, however, because babies are constantly growing and their caloric needs will change to accommodate their growth.

When it comes to feeding, changing, and managing two babies, especially while sleep deprived, life can get a bit foggy. Our advice to managing life with twins is to do everything for your babies at the same time, especially feedings.

MILK STORAGE

One surefire way of derailing your day as a new dad is having to pour a bottle of pumped breast milk or "liquid gold" down the drain. Now, while we know that you would *never* do such a thing, these milk storage guidelines will help you stay out of the doghouse for ruining perfectly good breast milk or wasting expensive formula.

Breast milk storage is simple if you remember the rule of six. Freshly pumped breast milk can be kept at room temperature for six hours, in the refrigerator for six days, or in a typical freezer for six months (12 months if you have a deep freezer). If you are tasked with thawing frozen breast milk just know that it must be consumed within 24 hours, cannot be refrozen, and should not be heated in a microwave.

Formula guidelines are relatively simple as well. Powder formula can be made in large batches using a pitcher with a mixing blade, like the Dr. Brown's formula pitcher, and kept in the refrigerator for use within 24 hours, while the ready-made kind, once opened, can be refrigerated and used within 48 hours.

REFLUX SUPPORT

The Mayo Clinic states that reflux or gastroesophageal reflux (GERD) affects one in five babies; twin parents will have a higher chance of a baby with reflux. Symptoms range from frequently spitting up milk to more severe abdominal discomfort, fussiness, and night waking. To put your mind at ease, reflux is rarely serious and generally improves as your baby gets older. In the meantime, to help make your babies more comfortable you can:

★ Do smaller, more frequent feedings.

★ Hold your baby upright after feedings (15 to 30 minutes).

★ Elevate your babies while they sleep.

★ Offer a pacifier after eating.

★ Burp your babies more often during feedings.

★ Use a hypoallergenic or gentle stomach formula.

HELPFUL GEAR AND HACKS

Feeding two babies can start to feel mundane when you do it a gazillion times a day. If there is one group of parents out there notoriously good at finding shortcuts, it's twin parents. Here are a few tricks to make double the feedings go a little more smoothly.

★ Invest in a TwinZ Pillow, Table for Two, or two Boppy pillows to help you bottle-feed two babies simultaneously.

★ While your partner is nursing, be nearby in case you need to help reposition a baby.

★ Have a few formula dispensing bottles (the kind that keep the formula and water separate until ready to mix) on hand to help simplify feeding on the go. Having extra bottles ready in our cars was helpful if we were out and about and needed a backup. You forget a lot in those early days.

★ Use a single-serving coffee maker instead of investing in a bottle warmer. Have the coffee machine dispense hot water into a cup or bowl. Soak a cold bottle of breast milk or formula and it's ready in three to five minutes.

★ Batch mix formula in a (formula-specific) pitcher and pre-make bottles for the entire day and night.

Documenting Memories

Before we had kids, when someone told us that "time flies" our eyes would roll with a "yeah, yeah, we know." Once our twins showed up, life suddenly hit fast-forward. Like most new parents, we filled our phones with adorable photos and videos. Documenting memories is what parents instinctively do; at least until your kids are old enough to be turning the eye roll on you.

Capturing them is the easy part. From the minute you walk into the hospital you will be snapping photos and videoing all the action. Before you know it, you won't know what to do with them all. Our goal in sharing this advice isn't to add one more stressor to your list of things to manage, but rather to help you keep them organized for the years to come.

Start by downloading a few photo apps that will do a lot of the heavy lifting for you. You want an app that will organize photos by your child's age, sync photos to all your devices, easily delete unwanted photos, share memories with your loved ones, and even create photo albums with a few quick clicks. Coming from two gals who haven't even created wedding albums, that's a big win.

Now, let's talk about video. It can easily take up all of your storage and then some. A word to the wise: back everything up to the cloud or another storage device.

Keeping videos organized isn't terribly hard, but it does require you to make a routine out of uploading and organizing them. Each month, put all the short video clips into an editing app. In a few short minutes you can throw together a monthly video that you can then upload to YouTube. A private YouTube account is a great place for your video management needs. Not to worry, YouTube allows you to text a link to your friends and loved ones so they can enjoy video memories of your kids that are otherwise hidden from the public.

The Gift of a Schedule

Becoming a dad of two babies suddenly lands you in uncharted waters. Once you set foot outside the hospital away from the all-knowing medical staff, it's on you to steer the ship. Hopefully you used your time surrounded by nurses, lactation consultants, and visitors to learn enough so your home life can mimic the routine established at the hospital.

Settling in at home is exciting—and overwhelming. Each time your head hits the pillow after surviving with two babies feels like a small victory. You're living by the eat-sleep-play-poop-repeat clock. If there is one piece of advice you should remember from this chapter it's this: a schedule and consistent routine will be the light at the end of your foggy, new-dad tunnel.

You might flip through these pages a time or two while a baby naps on your chest and think that we are crazy to even suggest setting up a schedule for two newborn babies. Your babies can't tell time, and let's be real, sleep deprivation affects your ability to use a clock too. Don't worry, we aren't referring to a schedule driven by time, but rather by specific routines repeated throughout the day.

In the beginning, while sleep develops and day versus night confusion is working itself out, a schedule is set by feeding, changing, and laying your babies down to sleep at the same time. As time goes on, your babies will spend more time awake, giving you the ability to add in some playtime to the routine.

In the first six to eight weeks with your babies, nail down consistent routines for feeding and sleeping. Create a tracking system to identify the patterns that form the foundation of your schedule. Either develop a printable spreadsheet of your own or head to CallistoMediaBooks.com/YouCanTwo to print out copies of our baby tracker, which will help you record every nap, bottle, or poopy diaper.

As the days pass and your hair turns a little grayer, age-appropriate awake times and feeding increments become more predictable. And as these patterns develop—adding in a little time to play—you will know when these things need to happen, thus allowing you to set a schedule.

Implementing a schedule doesn't have to be the be-all and end-all. It's not for everyone. With twins, scheduling forces you to be on your game. It can make life with two babies a lot easier than if you try to improvise each day, especially when you are sleep deprived. For your own sanity, we encourage you to try. It doesn't have to be extremely rigid, but with a little discipline and persistence your new normal might be easier than you think.

Twins Schedule Tracker Day/Date _____

Baby A

TIME	FEEDING	DIAPER
	_____ mins _____ ounces	bm _____ pee _____
	_____ mins _____ ounces	bm _____ pee _____
	_____ mins _____ ounces	bm _____ pee _____
	_____ mins _____ ounces	bm _____ pee _____

Baby B

TIME	FEEDING	DIAPER
	_____ mins _____ ounces	bm _____ pee _____
	_____ mins _____ ounces	bm _____ pee _____
	_____ mins _____ ounces	bm _____ pee _____
	_____ mins _____ ounces	bm _____ pee _____

Day/Date _____

Baby A

SLEEP TIME	DURATION	NOTES

Baby B

TIME	FEEDING	DIAPER

How to Do Everything for Two

Being a new dad is a lot to take in, especially when you are tasked with taking care of two babies at once, which makes the learning curve rather steep. For most new families, meeting the needs of one baby feels like a lot, but twin parents have that times two. If you don't have any other children, this will be all that you know. If you already have a child at home, well, then you already know what you are up against. When you are the only adult around, you have no choice but to figure out how to manage, and soon you'll realize how capable you really are. Until then, here are some tips.

HOW TO EASILY HOLD TWO BABIES AT ONCE

If you can carry two drinks down the crowded bleachers at a basketball game, carrying your newborn twins will be a breeze. Be sure there is support (pillows or a carrier) nearby to help you manage both babies at the same time. Use the football hold (keeping their heads closest to your body) or place them against your chest and cross your arms over them to hold them securely. We suggest that you take your first pass at this with others around, for safety reasons, before attempting it alone. Fortunately, carrying both of your twins at the same time will become easier as they get bigger and stronger.

HOW TO SWADDLE TWO BABIES

Place your twins on the floor or in their cribs. Prepare by laying both swaddles on a flat surface, folding the top edge of the blanket inward about six to eight inches. Your babies should be placed on the blankets with their necks lying on the fold. With each blanket, bring a corner across your baby's body and tuck it tightly underneath. Bring the bottom corner of the blanket up and tuck it in. Finally, wrap the last corner around your baby and snugly tuck the tail in. The swaddle should not be overly tight, but should be tight enough to ensure that your baby can't wiggle themselves out. It is easiest to fully swaddle one baby, move them back to the crib, then swaddle the second baby.

HOW TO FEED TWO BABIES AT ONCE

As dad, when it comes to feeding your twins simultaneously, you've got options. You'll need a TwinZ Pillow (our absolute favorite), Table for Two, or two Boppy pillows. Prepare, warm, and test the temperature of the milk on your wrists before feeding it to your babies. Once you're ready, lay both babies in the pillow in a reclining position. Simply bring the nipples of the bottles to their mouths and your babies will take it from there. If they struggle to get started, a few drops of milk on their lips generally does the trick.

HOW TO DOUBLE BURP

One of the coolest moves a twin dad can master is the *double burp*. You'll need to burp your babies throughout a feeding. The easiest way is to burp one baby at a time, but for the sake of time, try burping both babies at the same time. Remember when we talked about carrying your babies at the same time? This hold, where your arms are crossed over your chest where your babies are nestled, is the one you'll want to use. Pick your babies up, place them on your chest with their heads leaning over each shoulder, cross your arms, and firmly (yet gently) pat their backs.

HOW TO CALM TWO CRYING BABIES

Much like managing an emergency room full of trauma patients, as a twin dad you have to triage your babies' needs. Crying is a baby's way of communicating they need something, so the logical thing is to prioritize who needs what. It can feel overwhelming when your two babies are screaming and you're alone. Take a deep breath, then rule out injury or illness. Next, tend to the most obvious needs first, typically the baby who is in the most distress. The conundrum for twin parents is that often one baby is left crying until the needs of their sibling have been met, leaving parents feeling guilty or stressed. Remember that babies cry. You are only one set of hands and it's not likely you'll be able to fix everything for everyone at the same time. It may take a few minutes, but you will get both babies calm and happy again. Kick the self-doubt!

HOW TO GET OUT OF THE HOUSE WITHOUT YOUR PARTNER AS A NEW TWIN DAD

Getting out of the house as a new twin dad can feel intimidating at first, but getting out into the world does a lot for your mental health. Aside from preparedness, the key to surviving solo outings with your twins is flexibility. Parents with twins quickly learn to make the most of any situation that comes their way. When that first public blowout happens, don't panic. Like a great quarterback in a do-or-die playoff drive, you must rise to the occasion. And don't let derailed outings discourage you; chaos is par for the course. When all else fails, turn around, head home, and try again later after you've regrouped.

Think of everything you might need for your outing and then pack extra. Make a list; check it twice. Speaking from experience, there's nothing worse than having to use a paper towel from the bathroom as a makeshift diaper. Pack a diaper bag full of everything you could possibly need. The general rule is to leave the house for short errands with clean diapers and full tummies so that everyone is as happy as possible, you included. Those first few outings are important confidence-building opportunities for you to get comfortable getting out of the house. You don't need to be a champ on the first try.

> *Meghan:* When our boys were only four weeks old we decided to take a day trip for my husband's birthday. We tried our best to coordinate our drive around feedings and sleep, but boy oh boy were we in for an adventure. The car ride was filled with so many stops, pulling over to change diapers in the front seat of the car and feeding babies in gas station parking lots. Yes, I said gas stations! When we got there, we had lunch and a quick celebratory beer then got back in the car for the trek home, finally returning at 8:45 that night. We were gone for 12 hours yet seemed to accomplish very little. But hey, it was a great time for us as a couple to have good conversation and connect during the drive while we figured out our new normal.

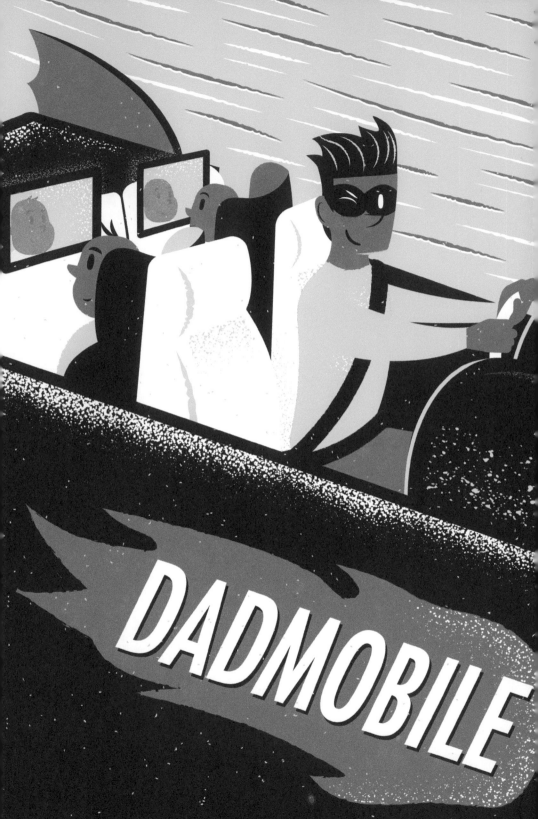

CHAPTER FIVE

THREE TO SIX MONTHS

By this point the rubber has met the road and you can confidently say that you have some twin parenting experience under your belt. Our hope is that your babies are plumping up, eating well, and minimizing blowouts. You're finding your groove, and big things are in store for the months to come. Sleep will become more consolidated and more predictable, while smiles, giggles, and growing personalities will tug on your heart. Parenting becomes wildly surreal (and maybe a bit cruel) when you begin to see glimpses of yourself in your children.

You have likely already gone back to work, but now is generally the time when your partner may be preparing to do the same and your babies will be adjusting to day care or a caretaker other than you or your partner. The big transitions don't slow down for a while. Many more firsts are yet to come. Continue to soak it all in but remember to take care of yourself and help your partner. As you tackle each new stage of parenting, be each other's compass. If you slide off course, readjust and get back on the road. As you gain experience remember to learn from it, both the wins and fails.

Milestones

Think about what your babies were like shortly after birth and compare that to what they have become after only a few months. Their growth and development are shocking. They quickly turn from sleepy swaddled burritos into social beings learning about the world around them. For those dads who struggled to bond with their babies after birth, these months will be a time when they may begin to feel a deeper connection with their babies. These milestones as defined by the CDC will help you track your babies' development at this age.

SOCIAL AND EMOTIONAL

Now is the time to get on the floor, roll up your sleeves, and play with your babies. They are beginning to develop a relationship with you. They can read your facial expressions, responding when you show them that you are happy, sad, or frustrated. As they reach four and five months, babies will begin to show excitement by laughing, squealing, and kicking their legs. They will typically show a lot of enjoyment because of the reactions they get from smiling and interacting with you and strangers. You'll get a lot of great moments too as you watch your babies absolutely delight someone.

VISUAL AND HEARING

If you haven't already, start chatting with your twins. Your babies are curious about the world around them. You will notice that they begin to watch people and objects, following them with their eyes, even at farther distances. Grabbing and putting objects in their mouths helps babies learn about objects in their world. As your babies pick things up, make a habit of naming things in single words to develop their vocabulary. Over the next several months your babies will learn to talk, beginning with small sounds. Imitating the sounds your babies make is the beginning of a conversation between you and them. These conversations help a baby to learn that they are separate from you and that language is how you connect to one another.

MOVEMENT AND PHYSICAL DEVELOPMENT

Babies, especially as they approach their half-birthday, become much more active. Over the course of the next three months, your babies' motor skills will change drastically. Keeping in mind that babies develop at different rates, typically you will begin to see your babies:

★ Roll over from their back to their belly and back again (four to six months)

★ Lift their head, chest, and arms during tummy time (four months)

★ Discover their hands and put them into their mouths often (three to four months)

★ Hold and play with toys on their back (four to five months)

★ Sit up while being held or on their own for a short time (around five months)

★ Grab for toys, objects, hair, and glasses (around five months)

★ Support their body weight when they are held up standing on their feet (around 8 months)

Remember this is a time when milestones can start to stress you out. If your doctor isn't worried, you shouldn't be either.

Medical Schedule

Thankfully, you've had a short break from continual doctor's appointments. After the two-month checkup, your babies' well-check schedule begins to slow down a bit.

By now you have hopefully had the experience of getting out and about with your twins alone so you can understand the challenge of taking two babies to the doctor without help. If you can, make it a practice to continue going with your partner to the doctor's appointments. Chances are, getting to the exam room with two babies in tow will have a few hiccups. The bombs of hunger and blown-out diapers always drop at the most inopportune times. There is a lot going on at these appointments, so an even ratio of parent to child generally eases everyone's stress. According to WhatToExpect.com, here's what you can expect from your babies' four-month and six-month visits.

FOUR-MONTH VISIT

Aside from the typical exam, you can expect your babies to receive the second dose of their rotavirus (RV), Tdap, Hib, PCV, and IPV vaccines, the first round of which they received at their two-month checkup. They should also have a hematocrit or hemoglobin screening to check for anemia.

SIX-MONTH VISIT

At your babies' half-birthday well-check, they will receive the third round of Dtap, PCV, and possibly Hib. Between now and 19 months they will need the third dose of IPV and hep B. At six months old, babies can get a flu shot (typically administered in two doses), which is a yearly recommendation during flu season. The doctor may do a TB test and check your babies' oral health, as their first teeth can show up as early as six months old.

Sleeping

Like fine wine, sleep gets better with age. During the three-to-six-month window, according to The Baby Sleep Site, you can expect your twins to sleep 15 to 16 hours in a 24-hour period between naps and night-time. Typically, by four months, you will begin to see more of a regular sleep and waking pattern, with many babies dropping the majority of their nighttime feedings. Keep in mind that every baby is on a different developmental schedule. Some babies will begin to take two to three longer naps, while others will stick to short naps. Some babies will sleep 12 hours a night without needing to eat, and other babies will still wake to eat regularly. Everything is highly dependent on each individual baby.

At this point, there are many parents who are satisfied with their twins' sleeping habits, and many others who are desperate for everyone to get more sleep. Here's pertinent sleep-related information for whichever camp you find yourself in.

SLEEP SCHEDULES

Up until now, knowing when your babies are tired has been highly dependent on their sleep cues (yawning, rubbing their eyes, etc.). As you move forward, in order to help develop and regulate their sleep patterns, you will want to establish regular bedtimes and naptimes that work for your family. Simply pick a time and stick to it as best as you can. If 7:00 p.m. is bedtime, you'll need to start your routine ahead of time so you have laid them down and asleep by 7:00 p.m. On the flip side, if you find that your babies are "sleeping in" past their typical morning wake time, wake them both up. It seems crazy and counterintuitive, but it will help them set their internal clock.

Your nap schedules can follow the clock, or you can choose to use age-appropriate awake windows to help you determine when naps should happen throughout the day. Either approach is appropriate as long as your babies are offered enough opportunities to sleep throughout the day. Naptime with twins can feel chaotic during these months. Around six months it will get easier and you will be able to work with their schedules to synchronize their daytime sleep.

From our own experiences and in working with twin families, it isn't uncommon for parents with two to feel like there is always one baby awake. This is where providing basic care at the same time helps synchronize their schedules. Laying your babies down to sleep, getting them up from sleep, and using bedtime routines will get your duo get adjusted and in sync, especially when one twin isn't quite as ready to rest.

SWADDLES

Swaddles are extremely helpful sleep tools for newborns, but most babies are usually ready to transition away from the swaddle and into a sleep sack around four months. Don't be shocked, though, if your babies use swaddles for a bit longer (even up to a year). The general rule is that swaddles are safe until your babies start rolling onto their tummies in their sleep. Although rolling can happen around three to four months, the motor skills required to roll without the use of their arms won't show up until closer to six months.

To begin the transition away from a swaddle, test the waters slowly. During a nap, swaddle your baby leaving one arm out. If that nap goes off without a hitch (they fall asleep and stay asleep), try another nap leaving both arms unswaddled. If your two-hour napper suddenly naps for 30 minutes with one arm free, go back to using the swaddle and try again in a few weeks.

> *Jenn:* It didn't take long before I realized that one of my boys loved the comfort of a swaddle and the other couldn't wait to bust out of it! I am still amazed every day that my kids are the same age yet have completely different preferences. One 2:00 a.m. feeding is all it took for me to realize that my son needed to transition into a sleep sack. I woke up to find him sleeping with his arms out. We immediately put him in a sleep sack and swaddled his brother for several more months.

SLEEP REGRESSIONS

With any luck things are just beginning to settle, your babies are beginning to sleep longer stretches at night, and that's when Mother Nature plays a mean joke on exhausted parents. Let us introduce you to sleep regressions. As described by Nicole Johnson, founder of The Baby Sleep Site, there are several points over the first two years of life (4, 8 to 10, 12, 18, and 24 months, give or take) when your babies may experience sleep regressions thanks to their cognitive and physical development.

FOUR-MONTH SLEEP REGRESSION

Around the four-month mark, your babies are sleeping less like new-borns and are beginning to sleep more like adults, spending less time in active sleep. You can expect fussiness, frequent nighttime wakings, and short naps. Focus on getting your babies down to sleep within age-appropriate awake time windows to avoid overtiredness, especially while you work through this regression.

You've heard it once, and we'll say it again: Your twins are two different people developing at different rates. That means there's no guarantee that your twins will experience a regression at the same time. You may need to prepare for overlapping regressions or they may occur back-to-back. When one regresses, you need to try your best and keep your regressor relatively on track while continuing to keep your other baby's healthy sleep habits and routines intact. Whatever you do, be consistent—keep naps and bedtimes the same. Temporary separations are not uncommon for twins' families; just be sure to mimic the sleep environment (dark and full of white noise) to make this transition smoother for everyone.

Although frustrating, sleep regressions are short lived, generally lasting a week or two. What you want to avoid is putting a Band-Aid on the problem. Small adjustments to get your waking babies back to sleep can quickly become bad habits and wreak havoc on your peaceful nights after a sleep regression has passed.

Feeding

Here's an area where things don't change much for another few months. You're welcome! Breast milk, formula, or a combination of both is all your babies will need. Over these short months your babies have become more efficient eaters and their stomachs have grown significantly in size, now being able to go three to four hours between feedings. Keep in mind that breastfeeding babies may need to eat sooner or more often. Most health care providers do not recommend that parents offer solid foods to babies younger than six months. So, sit back and enjoy these months, because things are about to get messy.

Feeding Chart

AGE	OUNCES PER FEEDING	NUMBER OF FEEDINGS IN 24 HOURS	HOURS BETWEEN FEEDINGS
1 month	2 to 4 ounces	8 to 10 feedings	1.5 to 3
2 months	5 to 6 ounces	8 to 10 feedings	2.5 to 3
3 to 5 months	6 to 7 ounces	8 to 9 feedings	3 to 4

Source: HerCottage.com

CHOOSING THE RIGHT NIPPLE

Get to know all that you can about nipples. No, really, we aren't kidding or being inappropriate. It is important to know what size nipples you're using and when to upgrade to a higher level. Many bottle brands offer nipple levels that correlate to a babies' age, generally ranging from preemie to level four.

Preemie or level one nipples are great options for breastfeeding babies who are going between the breast and bottle. The slower flow helps mimic the flow of their mother's nipple.

There isn't an absolute when it comes to changing nipples. Look for the following cues to determine if a particular nipple's flow isn't fast enough:

★ The babies begin to take longer to eat.

★ The babies are becoming fussy or agitated during a feeding.

★ The babies fall asleep.

If your babies need a slower-flow nipple you might see:

★ Gulping or hard swallowing

★ Coughing

★ Choking

★ Bottle refusal

★ Milk overflowing from their mouth

GROWTH SPURTS

Growth spurts happen a lot in the first year, and you're dealing with two babies who will likely be going through these phases at different times. In one year, according to KellyMom.com, your babies will likely go through seven different growth spurts, namely in the first few days after birth, at 7 to 10 days, at 2 to 3 weeks, at 4 to 6 weeks, and then at 3, 4, 6, and 9 months, give or take. When your babies are fussy and demanding more food, it's likely a growth spurt. They'll want to eat more often and consume larger amounts of milk than usual. During this time, the best thing you can do is follow your babies' lead, offering the breast or bottle as often as they demand.

A NOTE ABOUT BREASTFEEDING

Breastfeeding is different for every twin mom. Some thrive right away, others struggle from the get-go but continue to push through the challenges. There may come a time (if it hasn't come already) when your partner will choose to stop breastfeeding. Your job here is to provide support, empathy, and understanding. Your instinct may be to try to solve the problem and offer solutions, but tread lightly. Many women feel guilty because they need to stop nursing. They may be disappointed that they can't produce more milk, frustrated with pumping a million times a day, or just really want to wear a shirt again. Whatever your partner's reasoning, remember to be supportive and encouraging. It's likely that the end of her breastfeeding journey will be an emotional decision.

Cloth vs. Disposable Diapers

As newborns, a single baby will go through 10 to 12 diapers a day. That's about 320 diapers a month. Because you have *two* babies, you'll be changing around 640 diapers a month. Luckily after about the first month, babies use a few less diapers a day, closer to 8 rather than 10. That's a silver lining, right? Changing over 600 diapers a month can put a strain on your pocketbook, which is why it's important to know the benefits and drawbacks of cloth diapers vs. the disposable kind.

Diapers are a part of your life for a number of years. And with twins, you'll be a diaper-changing master after a few poops. Make things easier on yourself by setting up diaper changing stations in multiple rooms and on multiple floors around your home. Also, use legitimate diaper pails in these makeshift stations because you don't want those stinky diapers in your kitchen trash.

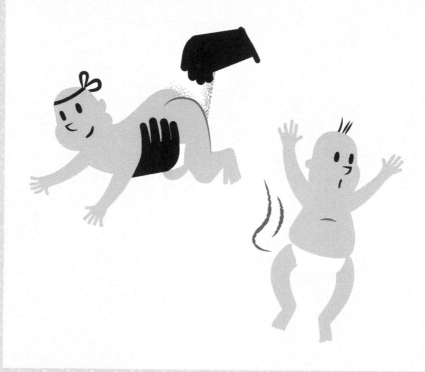

CLOTH DIAPERS	DISPOSABLE DIAPERS
A more cost-effective approach, costing around $800 to $1,000 per baby for two years.	Cost is heavier, ranging from $2,000 to $3,000 per baby for two years.
Reusable, making them ecofriendly. Can be reused on additional siblings that may come in the future.	A convenient option for busy parents of twins because you can toss them when you are done.
Gentler on sensitive skin.	Dyes and gels can irritate a baby's skin. You may have to try a variety of brands to find one that works for your babies.
Requires parents to scoop the poop into the toilet to clean. Electricity and water used to clean. Laundering services are available for a monthly fee.	Harsher on the environment. Dirty diapers in landfills can contaminate local water systems.
Have to be changed more often because they are generally less absorbent.	Unopened packages of diapers can be exchanged for larger sizes as your babies grow.
Most diaper rash creams or ointments can't be used with cloth diapers. They cause buildup on the diaper, affecting its absorbency.	Convenient when out and about or traveling because you don't have to carry dirty diapers around until you get home.

Source: TheBump.com

Travel

Put your big boy pants on, pack up, and go! Although traveling with your crew might seem like an overwhelming task at first, we are here to assure you that it is doable and actually enjoyable. New parents are exhausted and up to their elbows in poop, having gone days without a shower. All that can take a toll, which is why getting out into the real world, enjoying things that used to bring you joy, pre-kids, is essential to your well-being and your relationship. So, whether you hit the road or fly across the world, a few simple tips coupled with thoughtful preparation will make traveling with your twins something you can easily conquer.

Between our two families, we've taken countless trips, both on the road and in the air, and lived to tell about it. There have been blunders, delays, mid-flight blowouts, projectile vomiting, and toddlers licking the airplane. With all of that, not only did we survive, but we have learned a thing or two along the way. Our biggest piece of advice is to put some thought into your travel and remain extraordinarily flexible. Whether you are driving or flying, plan around naps and feedings. Choosing a flight that takes off at the witching hour will not set your travel plans up for success. Instead, aim for departure times that coincide with your babies' typical naptimes (say 9:00 a.m. and 1:00 p.m.). Although you cannot plan for everything that might happen on your adventure, you can do your best to keep things on track with your scheduling and preparation.

Once you've nailed down the best day and time to travel, packing should become your priority. Children, babies especially, require stuff. Lots and lots of stuff. As you begin your preparations, you'll want to think about the things your babies will need, the basics for you, and then an arsenal of extras to have on hand in the event that something goes awry . . . which it almost certainly will. Aside from these, think about everything you might need within a moment's notice to clean up any mess (we're talking poopy explosions and vomit), feed hungry bellies, or keep little babies entertained and happy. Organize your luggage so that hand sanitizer, wallets, and phones are easily accessible, always pack extra shirts, and keep the "nice to haves" to a minimum.

Flying with infants introduces a bit of an added challenge to traveling, but like we said, it isn't impossible. Be prepared to spend extra time at airport security while your breast milk bottles or sealed water bottles for mixing formula are screened. Consider preparing treat baggies with chocolates, candies, lip balm, and travel-size hand lotions for the flight attendants. A small gesture of kindness goes a long way, especially when toting two small babies onto a crowded airplane. By the time you are settled into your seats, the attendants at the back of the plane will already know that two cute babies are on board. This gesture tends to encourage flight attendants and fellow passengers to be more empathetic and understanding if your babies are having meltdowns. Someone might even offer to hold a baby to give you a much-needed break. We've even been surprised with freshly poured cocktails (with lids!) and snacks as a result of our treat bags.

Meghan: When my boys were five months old, we decided to fly to California so they could meet their great-grandparents. My anxiety increased at the thought of being stuck in an airplane for a few hours with two infants. I always considered myself a seasoned traveler, but traveling with my twins overwhelmed me thanks to so many unknowns. After our first voyage in the sky I realized that 1) I will never see these people again, 2) it's okay if my kids cry, and 3) being prepared saved me when the unexpected happened. I learned to roll with it all: the good, the bad, and everything in between.

Bathing

Every twin parent worries about managing things like bath time solo, and as two fellow twin parents, we are here to tell you that you are not alone. Managing multiple infants around water is anxiety producing for all parents. Thankfully, with practice, bathing two babies with only one set of hands can be safely done. When you find yourself staring down bath time with two babies and only one of you, know that you can absolutely handle it. Just be sure that water safety is your number one priority; never leave your babies unattended in or near the water.

SET UP AHEAD OF TIME

Getting things set up ahead of time is key so that when those babies get out of the tub, you have everything you need at arm's reach. Before you turn on the water, grab pajamas, diapers, butt creams, lotions, and towels. We find it helpful to bring a playmat or baby lounger into the bathroom to lay one baby down while you bathe and change the other.

BATH TIME HACK

Until your babies are old enough to sit up on their own, bathing them individually is generally the easier and safer route. Once they are sitting and stable, a plastic laundry basket is a great bath time tool to keep them contained in your tub without sliding around.

Self-Care for Dad

Your job, and likely the reason you are reading this book, is to be a supportive partner and help in caring for your new babies. But all that can wear a guy out. If you haven't already experienced it, there will be a long, exhausting night when neither baby will stop crying and you catch yourself being snappy toward your partner. Emotional and mental exhaustion comes in many forms, and when it does, it's a cue to take time for yourself. Parenting is hard; it can cause us to doubt ourselves and leave us feeling deflated at times.

Golf outings, game nights, or grabbing beers with a buddy were once an important part of your identity before your twins came along. Just because you have added "supportive partner" and "dad" to your résumé doesn't mean you need to stop doing those other things. One of the most important things new parents should do is make time for themselves and their relationship. We aren't saying go take multiple weekend-long guy trips, but deliberately carving out a few minutes each day or planning a happy hour every once in a while will have a positive impact; you'll return clearheaded and energized. The saying "absence makes the heart grow fonder" still rings true even if you are only away for a short while. Even getting something on the calendar to look forward to can make a big difference; knowing a planned break is coming is extremely comforting.

Self-care can take on many forms, and it doesn't always have to mean you are spending hours away from your family. It's all in your perspective, really. One powerful yet simple act of self-care can take only 15 minutes of your day.

★ Get up early and take the dog for a walk.

★ Take an extra-long bathroom break.

★ Use the sauna at the gym for 15 minutes after your workout.

★ Grab a coffee or a beer with someone.

★ Get a haircut or beard trim.

★ Take a long, hot shower.

★ Make something in the garage after bedtime.

★ Read a book.

★ Journal.

★ Commit to a clean eating plan.

★ Have a cocktail by the fire after bedtime.

A Supportive Note from Our Husbands: Somewhere along the way, in your new role, you will hit a wall. It might not be that dramatic, but there will come a time when you will be overwhelmed—physically, emotionally, or both. It's okay because it happens to everyone. Your sleep isn't the same as it was before your twins arrived, and when you do get some, it's not the same. You may turn into a light sleeper, waking up at the sound of a pin drop, or the opposite may occur, where you [can] sleep through an earthquake because you are so exhausted. Remember that you have two very different babies to tend to and this first year will be tough at times. Our advice to you is to take a step back, look at things from a bird's-eye view, and allow yourself a little leeway to be less than your best. Remember to take care of yourself too. Newsflash: You're the backbone of this operation. Your family needs you now more than ever. So, do what you need to do to survive in the moment, then get back in the game.

Meghan: As much as feeding your babies is a necessity, feeding yourself is too. If you asked my husband about ways he cared for himself when our babies were young, [he] would tell you that he focused on eating well for himself. If there was ever a time in his life that he dialed in his eating habits, it was after our kids were born. He didn't have time to feel sluggish after a meal. We were up all hours at night and busy trying to keep up with our busy day-to-day responsibilities. The last thing he wanted was to be in a food coma. Make yourself a priority alongside the rest of the family. Can you have the occasional pizza and beer? You bet! But overall, eat the best you can when you can. You'll thank yourself later.

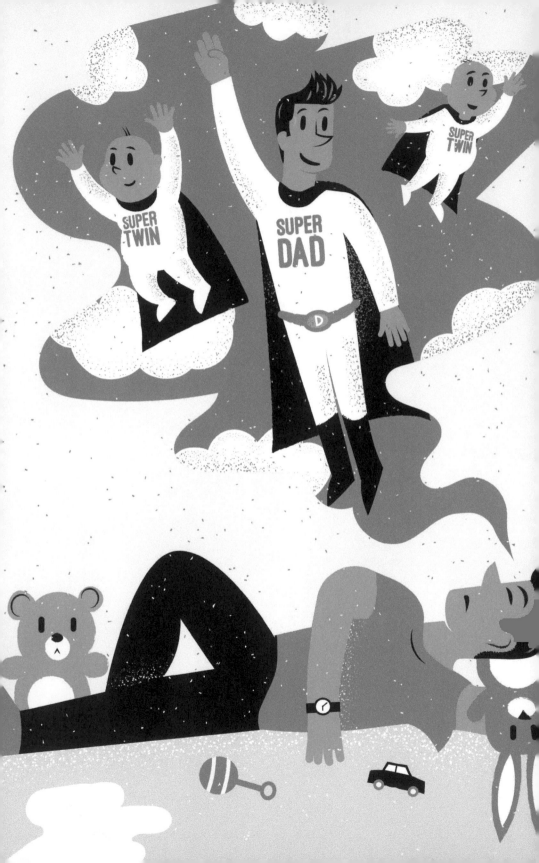

CHAPTER SIX

SIX TO NINE MONTHS

Have you looked in the mirror lately? When you spend most of your time bouncing and lugging around two babies, twin dads get ripped. You've made it halfway to your twins' first birthday, and as you turn the corner to the second half of this monumental year, we hope you're feeling a little less tired. Over the next few months, parenting will take a slight turn because your babies will become more active participants in your family's life.

You will begin to notice your babies observing their surroundings, watching your every move, taking an interest in your food, and babbling up a storm. They may be sitting up and possibly becoming mobile (Gasp! We cover babyproofing later, don't worry.), and they're ready to start eating solid foods. This can feel like a lot to tackle, but you have nothing to worry about because we cover it all in this chapter. These few months are also a time to really enjoy and embrace the change because your twins are one step closer to toddlerhood, which is a mess of fun all in itself.

Milestones

Along the way you will find yourself thinking, "This is the best stage yet!" Then a new phase comes along and it gets even better; there are so many crazy moments in parenting that arise unexpectedly. Your babies are changing daily and their personalities are booming. Their bond as twins is developing. You get to watch two very different, but uniquely connected, humans coexist and begin to participate in the world around them. You will see your twins becoming more aware of each other, and you get to witness moments where they hold hands, make each other laugh, and even practice sharing with one another. As a parent you'll morph from a spectator to an active participant who is now herding two busy (pint-size) people. The milestones below, as established by the CDC, will help you track all the exciting developments to come at this age.

SOCIAL AND EMOTIONAL

Between six and nine months, there are some big emotional changes. In these months, your twins will come to understand that they are separate from you (and their twin sibling) with feelings of their own that they are learning to process and exert. They will begin to communicate their needs more explicitly. The first of many parent-child clashes may begin now. They will become increasingly more comfortable with familiar people in their world, making "stranger danger" more apparent.

VISUAL AND HEARING

As your babies' eyes strengthen, they will be able to focus on smaller objects. They develop depth perception and you'll notice they become aware of heights and falling. Don't be surprised when your babies spend more time talking or screaming and enjoy making lots of noise with any tools they can get their hands on. Now is the time to hide your pots, pans, and spatulas!

MOVEMENT AND PHYSICAL DEVELOPMENT

If they haven't already, within the next few months your twins will most likely sit up for longer periods without assistance. Babies' movement can land anywhere on the spectrum from scooting to crawling too fast to catch. They will start to move objects from one hand to the other and might even pick something up if it is dropped on the floor. You might hear your first babbles and you'll lose your mind. It doesn't get any cuter than that.

Medical Schedule

Now that they aren't making monthly appearances at the pediatrician's office, parents typically shift their energy to keeping kids out of a doctor's office until the next well-check. At some point within the first year, as we all muddle through the cold and flu season, illness will likely strike. When babies get sick, it stinks. When two babies get sick at the same time, it really stinks. And if you walk into that nine-month well-check appointment still free of experiencing that first illness, hats off to you. This month's well-check appointment isn't much different from the others, with a physical and oral examination, a discussion of milestones, and the final doses of IPV and hep B immunizations (which can be given anywhere between now and 18 months). Per usual, if it is cold and flu season, your pediatrician will recommend a flu shot for your babies after six months of age.

SURVIVING SHOTS

Soothing babies is the name of the game after they get a round of shots at the doctor. Although pediatric nurses work wonders to make things as quick and painless as possible, getting shots, especially more than one, is just no fun. If your babies are due for vaccines, have two bottles ready or plan to stay and nurse them immediately afterward. Take your time when leaving the doctor's office after these appointments and know that you never need to rush out of the door. Everyone, including you, deserves a minute to regroup before moving on with the day.

The Terror of Teething

Excessive drool and an obsession with gnawing on everything in sight can only mean one thing . . . your babies' teeth are about to make their debut. When it comes to teething, remember all babies are different. Chances are, your twins will be very different teethers, getting their teeth at very different times. According to WebMD, teeth start showing up anywhere from four to seven months and will continue coming in until around 24 months. Some babies will exhibit all of the classic teething symptoms while others will stoically manage until you suddenly discover that they have two front teeth. Do your best to recognize their discomfort and find ways to provide them some relief.

Symptoms of Teething:

★ Bringing hands and other objects to their mouth

★ Excessive drooling

★ Excessive fussiness

★ Interrupted sleep patterns

★ Low-grade temperature

★ Rash around the mouth

★ Refusal to eat solids

Ways to Alleviate Pain:

★ Breastfeeding. Not only is nursing a soothing activity for your baby, but breast milk has healing properties.

★ Offer chilled puréed fruits (if your babies are eating solids).

★ Freeze washcloths, plastic teething rings, or spoons and allow your babies to gnaw on them.

★ Frozen fruit inside mesh teethers. Just be sure to wipe their gums afterward to help prevent tooth decay.

★ Give them a gum massage by gently rubbing their gums with your clean finger.

★ Offer homemade popsicles to gnaw on.

★ Medications like numbing gels or creams or homeopathic teething tablets are not recommended for infants. Avoid anything that uses benzocaine, as it can be potentially fatal if swallowed.

★ Over-the-counter pain medication. When all else fails and nothing seems to be easing their pain, talk with your child's doctor about using infant Tylenol (acetaminophen) or ibuprofen. Suppositories seem icky but can be a lifesaver if your baby resists taking medicine.

Meghan: Teething happens when you least expect it. Neither of our twins were symptomatic teethers in the same way, which made it hard to know what was actually happening. While we were on a family vacation, one of our boys was uncharacteristically fussy with a low-grade fever and incessant drool. We wondered if he caught a bug on the plane. New parents here, we had no clue! After a long night of crying, we woke up to new teeth; my grandma noticed his bloody gums! Blame it on fatigue or just being a new parent, but we had no idea that he was teething. To help everyone manage while on vacation, we took a lot of walks outdoors, gave him cold washcloths to suck on, and did our best to keep him comfortable. On the flip side, when our other twin broke his first tooth he showed no noticeable signs, which was just a reminder to us that they will always experience life differently.

Creating Healthy Sleep Habits

Sleep is something that all parents could use more of, and we have yet to work with a family that wants less of it. Since babies aren't inherently born knowing how to be champion sleepers, you have to teach them. Teaching your babies healthy sleep habits improves the well-being of your entire family. Stanford's Children's Health says:

★ Sleep is important for the maturation of a baby's brain.

★ A lack of sleep has been linked to developmental delays and obesity.

★ Well-rested babies have a calmer temperament and are more adaptable.

★ Sleep deprivation puts mothers at higher risk for postpartum depression.

Sleep is a basic human need. While it is nice to think, "this is only a phase," or "I might as well just soak up this time with my babies," there is a reason why you need to teach your babies to be good, independent sleepers. We've been in your shoes and get that sleep deprivation sucks. It can start to affect every part of your life. Unfortunately, sleepless months are a natural part of parenting, and with twins, it is a little bit harder at times. When your babies are ready to sleep through the night—once they've doubled their birth weight and can consume at least 24 ounces in a 24-hour period—you'll need to get your game face on. You need to mentally and physically prepare to teach healthy sleep habits to your babies while you power through the challenges that will come your way in the middle of the night.

Ready to do this? To begin, develop and implement a bedtime routine. The steps included in your routine are not as important as the consistency with which you follow that pattern of steps *every single night*. A solid bedtime routine is a great foundation to lay before helping your babies to learn to sleep through the night.

As early as possible (after about six weeks, of course), begin teaching your babies to fall asleep *independently*. Lay them down in a *very* drowsy state, but with their eyes still open slightly. Call us crazy, we know what you're thinking. Your babies have been falling asleep at every feeding, so laying them down awake is downright impossible. It can be done. When they're about to fall asleep, wake them just enough to see the whites of their eyes before laying them down.

The ability to fall asleep independently is a vital component to teaching your babies to sleep. It can be more challenging for your babies to learn as they get used to any "props," such as pacifiers, rocking, feeding to sleep, or anything given or used to help your babies fall asleep. The earlier you break a dependence, the easier it will be to teach your twins to sleep through the night. On that note, let's discuss sleep associations.

SLEEP ASSOCIATIONS

Your bedtime routine and the supports that you have provided are what your babies will associate with sleep and what will help them independently fall back to sleep when they wake. Props that help your babies fall asleep aren't necessarily problematic until your babies cannot fall asleep without them. Spending countless hours at night rocking or replacing binkies becomes a problem because your babies aren't falling asleep or staying asleep without your intervention. You want to find ways to provide comfort to your babies that doesn't keep everyone up all night long. If you continue to go back in the room every time your babies cry because they're tossing their pacifiers out of the crib, nobody gets any sleep. Instead, try looking for tools that promote self-soothing, like white noise machines or lovies.

> *Jenn:* Not long after our twins were born, sleep deprivation, hormonal shifts, and a general sense of inadequacy took its toll on me. It was suggested to us to hire a postpartum doula specializing in multiples. She taught me all the tricks of the trade and ended up being a lifesaver. At one point she told me to stuff my bra with these little square lovies that we were gifted at a baby shower. After [I wore] those around for a few hours, she laid our babies down for

a nap [with the lovies] and they miraculously fell asleep. The lovies absorbed my scent and helped comfort my boys in my absence. Lesson learned here: Accept help and be open to trying something new.

SLEEP ENVIRONMENT

Do you like the room cooler with all the lights off? What happens if you get too hot in the middle of the night? You wake up, right? Similarly, the environment where your babies sleep has an impact on their ability to fall asleep and stay asleep throughout the night.

★ **Temperature.** According to SleepAdvisor.org, the nursery should ideally be kept at 68 to 72 degrees Fahrenheit, allowing you to dress your twins in one layer of pajamas and a sleep sack or swaddle.

★ **White noise.** White noise machines simulate the comforts of the womb, which was a noisy place. The noise can be a soothing constant that will help lull the babies back to sleep if they wake. It also helps offset any sudden noises, like an Amazon delivery that just had to show up once they went down for a nap.

★ **Transitional objects.** You want restful sleep for the entire family, which means that you need to teach your babies ways to soothe themselves without your assistance. No one wants to be up every hour replacing pacifiers that have been launched out of the crib. Transitional objects—like a small stuffed animal, a lovey, or a soft book—are helpful tools for soothing babies in your absence.

Feeding

Whether you are more of a takeout lover or a talented at-home chef, now is the time to get cooking so that you can introduce your twins to a variety of foods. Yes, 90 percent of what you serve your babies will end up on the floor or in their hair, but messy is fun, right? Pediatricians generally recommend introducing solids at six months of age, when your babies can sit upright with control of their head and neck, are taking an interest in what you are eating, and have lost the tongue thrust reflex that automatically pushes food out of their mouth. Are your babies seemingly hungry after a day's worth (32 ounces) of formula or breast milk? It may be time to add a meal of solid foods. Solids are in addition to the regimen of breast milk and formula that your babies are used to until their first birthday when you can then switch to whole milk.

As you begin offering solid foods, get out the camera because the facial expressions your babies will make as they try new flavors are priceless. The mess that goes along with this adventure is pretty fun to capture too!

For the first few months with solids, the majority of babies' calories and nutrition will still come from formula or breast milk. The goal of mealtimes in the beginning is creating a routine around eating rather than providing nutrition. While you introduce your babies to the tastes and textures of food, begin by adding one meal a day of one to two tablespoons, according to the CDC. Then work up to three meals with a serving the size of your baby's fist. By their first birthday you should have an eating schedule in place that includes three square meals and two snacks.

WHAT AND WHEN: INTRODUCING SOLIDS

You won't find a chart that tells you exactly which foods to introduce when. Typically, parents choose to start with iron-fortified cereal, mixed with breast milk or formula for a runny consistency. The CDC recommends adding in one new fruit, vegetable, or meat every three to five days to help identify any foods that may cause unwanted reactions. You can purée, mash, or chop soft finger foods (hard-boiled egg, cheese, cooked pasta, etc.), which your babies can begin pinching around eight months.

BABY-LED WEANING

There is a philosophy of feeding babies that doesn't require parents to purée or mash the food that is offered. Parents who adopt baby-led weaning offer their babies gummable foods (think avocado, tomato, peaches, bananas, etc.) in large pieces that babies can hold with their fists. The idea is to give babies the opportunity to feed themselves healthy foods that interest them right out of the gate, with the ability to control how much they put into their mouths. Offering whole, gummable foods allows babies to learn to chew first (or, more accurately, gum first) and swallow, and aids in their digestion.

A WORD ABOUT ALLERGIES

Introducing solids is a fun milestone, but reactions or aversions to foods makes parents a little on edge every time something new is offered. The American Academy of Pediatrics recommends that babies are introduced to high-allergen foods like eggs, nuts, and seafood early in the solid food journey, but no later than 11 months to reduce the chances of developing a food allergy.

After you have successfully introduced a few different foods, offer your babies those allergen foods one at a time, while at home. A reaction can include gas or diarrhea, rashes around the mouth and bottom, and vomiting. Watery eyes, fussiness, or wheezing are also considered signs of a reaction. If this happens to your little one, wait a week and try again. Unless you start to see swelling of the lips and face, or the wheezing intensifies: then it's time to call 911. If the reactions are mild, then three consecutive reactions will confirm a sensitivity to a particular food, but that doesn't necessarily mean you have to eliminate it forever. With the support of your pediatrician, wait a few months and try again.

ARE THERE THINGS TO AVOID?

The list isn't long, but there are things to avoid for the time being. Honey can be contaminated with bacteria that causes infant botulism and choking hazards like whole nuts and grapes are not recommended.

FOR THE CHEF

Many parents enjoy making their own baby food. This can be particularly cost effective for parents who have to feed two babies. A pot for steaming, a food processor, and a little creativity are all you need to open up a whole new world of flavors for your baby. In the beginning, stick to single-food recipes; later, you can get creative blending foods and spices (not salt or added sugar) together. A batch of purées can be stored in the freezer in silicone storage trays and defrosted at mealtime, helping save you a few bucks.

Babyproofing

With two babies becoming more mobile, it's time to tighten up the security around your home. As soon as they are crawling, look out! It's just the beginning. As twin parents you will notice how much they head in opposite directions, keeping you constantly on your toes. Before you know it, you'll have a roll of toilet paper strung across the living room while at the same time your pots and pans are being spread across the kitchen floor.

Learning to crawl gives your baby the expanded ability to explore their world. Their curiosity spikes, and they will begin getting into places that you don't want them to explore. The laundry room, under the kitchen sink, and the trash are all fair game. But what about not-so-obvious places like the poisonous plant at the base of your stairs? It's never too early to babyproof your pad. If possible, tackle this project early so that you aren't scrambling at the last minute. You can always adjust as your twins uncover ways to outsmart your babyproofing. All it takes is one curious baby to dismantle the TV remote to make you realize how many things you've missed.

One Amazon order will give you all the gear you need to get started. We suggest moving from room to room to evaluate the dangers that each space presents to your babies. Keep in mind that their vantage point is very different from your own; take the time to look at each room of your house from a variety of perspectives. Get down on the floor and observe your home from their level.

Babyproofing Checklist

LIVING AREAS	
☐	Cover all outlets.
☐	Install baby gates at the top and bottom of the stairs.
☐	Remove TV remotes with batteries from reach.
☐	Add foam bumpers to fireplaces, sharp corners, and coffee tables.
☐	Remove matches, lighters, and candles, or store them out of reach.
☐	Remove wobbly or unstable furniture for the time being.
☐	Remove or anchor large furniture, TVs, bookcases, etc.
☐	Install pinch guards on all the doors.
☐	Hide electrical cords.
☐	Secure electrical cords.

KITCHEN	☐ Put locks on all cabinets, especially under the sink.
	☐ Store toxic chemicals in a locked cabinet or somewhere out of reach.
	☐ Install a temperature guard on your water heater.
	☐ Install stove knob covers.
	☐ Move pet food and water out of reach.
	☐ Use the rear stove burners to cook.
NURSERY/ BEDROOMS	☐ Remove blinds with loop cords or install cord stops.
	☐ Cover all outlets.
	☐ Install safety guards on all windows.
	☐ Ensure that dressers and changing tables are secured to the wall.
	☐ Move other furniture away from the crib.
	☐ Store small toys in plastic containers or out of reach.
	☐ Take down decorative mobiles.

Babyproofing Checklist

BACKYARD	☐ Cover the grill.
	☐ Keep propane out of reach.
	☐ Cover basement well windows with metal grates.
	☐ Install a baby gate to deck stairs.
	☐ Install or evaluate the function of fences/gates. If you have a pool, a heavy-duty locked gate is an investment but a must.
GARAGE	☐ Relocate all toxic and dangerous chemicals out of reach and in a locked location.
	☐ Lock up all tools.
	☐ Add a lock to the door going in and out of the house.
	☐ Check that the garage door safety sensor is working properly.

BATHROOMS	☐ Install cabinet and toilet locks.
	☐ Lock up cleaning products or move out of reach.
	☐ Lock up prescriptions and medicines or move out of reach.
	☐ Move razors out of reach.
	☐ Remove or lock up bathroom trash cans.
	☐ Add faucet protectors to bathtub faucets.
LAUNDRY ROOM	☐ Babyproof the door handle.
	☐ Remove detergent pods from your home or lock them up. Liquid detergent is a safer alternative with children in your home.
	☐ Store iron in a locked closet.

Communicating with Sign Language

Communication barriers with your babies are without a doubt a frustrating part of parenting. If only they could talk to tell you how they felt. Great news! Now they can. Using infant sign language gives your twins the ability to communicate their needs far before they are able to use words. You can begin by simultaneously using signs while speaking with your babies. While some babies may begin signing back around six months, babies between eight and nine months have more hand control to use signs efficiently. Once your babies develop some basic sign vocabulary, communication becomes easier, easing frustration for everyone. As your babies gain confidence in communicating with you, seeing that their needs are understood and being met, their motivation grows to continue experimenting with language.

Babies learn from watching the adults around them. As you notice that your babies are taking an interest in communicating with you, begin using signs (making the hand gesture and saying the corresponding word) that are meaningful to your lifestyle.

It doesn't matter which signs you decide to incorporate as long as they help your children communicate their everyday needs. "Please," "thank you," "more," "hungry," "thirsty," and "tired" are great places to start, teaching manners right off the bat. The key to signing success is consistency, repetition, and instant gratification; your baby will learn best if they are promptly given what they have asked for. The intention here is to reduce frustration and make your interactions easier, so follow your babies' lead. Use their invented signs and be observant. Each of your twins will adapt to and use sign language differently; you might find one baby really taking to it while the other might not.

By no means do you have to become proficient in American Sign Language (ASL) to win here. Signing with babies is intended to be simple. Don't go overboard trying to learn a million signs, just use those that are helpful in communicating your babies' everyday needs. Be sure to include your partner and other caretakers so that everyone spending time with your babies is on the same page.

Sign Language Starter List

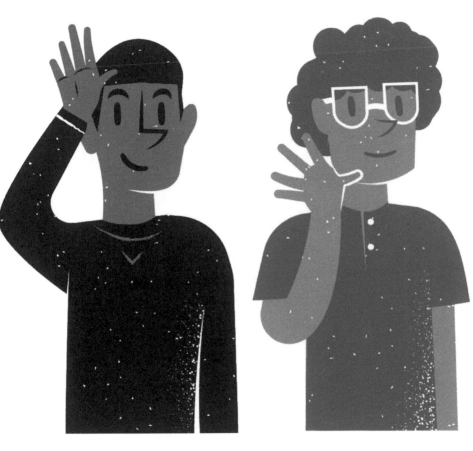

Dad   Mom

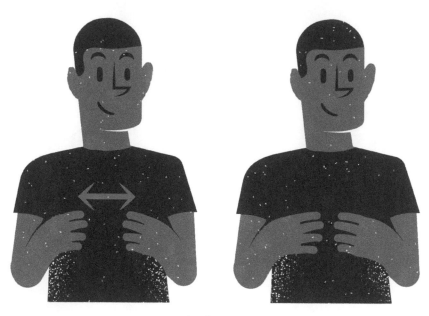

More

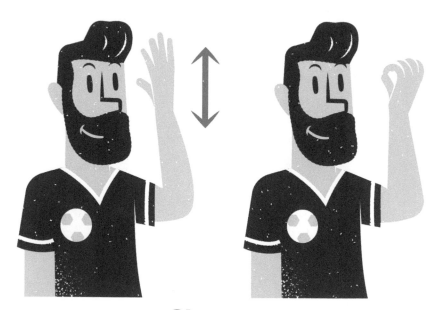

Sleepy

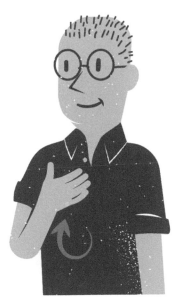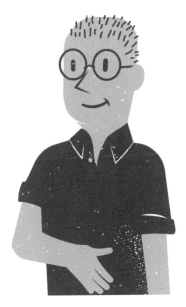

Please

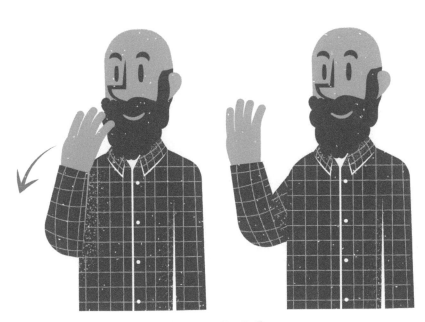

Thank You

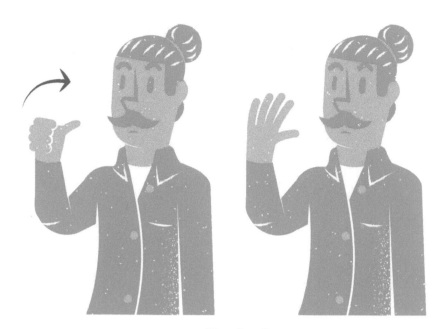

Drink

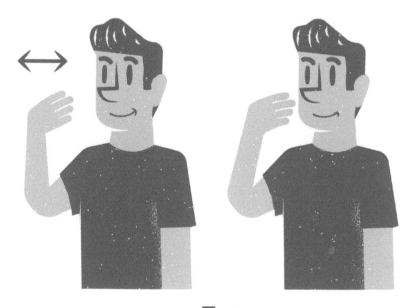

Eat

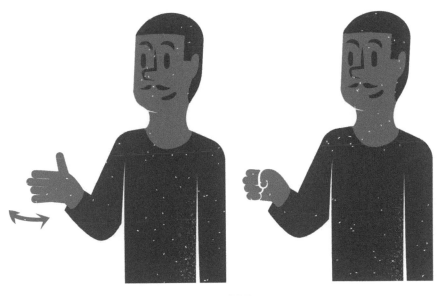

Milk

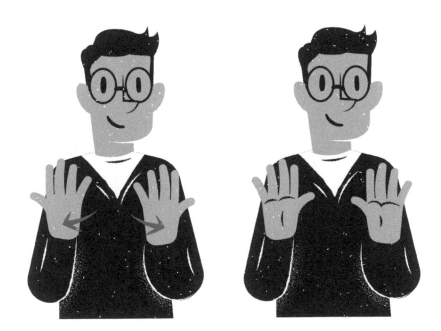

All Done

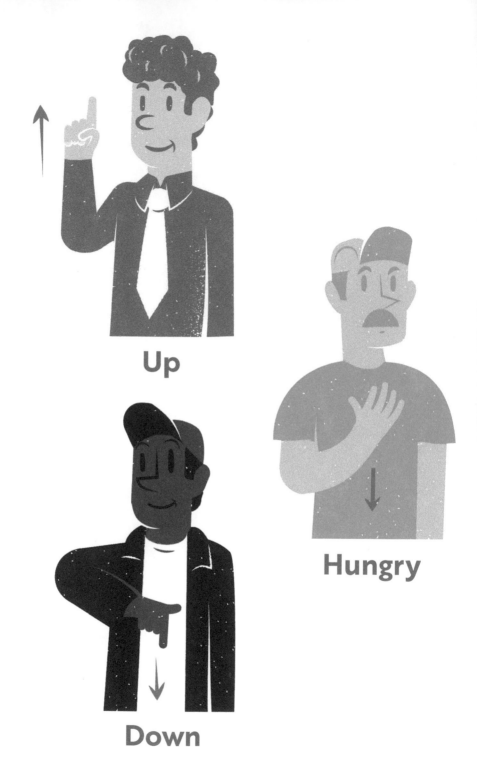

Up

Hungry

Down

Tackling Naps

If we had a dollar for every time a client asked us when their twins would finally nap at the same time, well, we'd be sipping mai tais on our private island right about now. It is the million-dollar question that has several answers. We get it. Being up with your infants at night is exhausting enough, which makes naptime an ideal moment for a parenting break. But what happens when one baby falls asleep for their morning nap and the other only dozes off right as the first sleeper wakes? You don't get a minute to yourself.

To some extent it won't matter how many routines and rituals you put into place or how diligent you are about being home for naptime, napping feels like a crapshoot. That is until around their half-birthday, when daytime sleep consolidates and naps lengthen. You read that right . . . longer, synchronized naps are on the horizon. Until then, shorter (by short we mean 20 to 120 minutes), slightly unpredictable naps are developmentally appropriate. As you begin to work on improving naptime with your twins, understand that it is a work in progress.

SEPARATE OR TOGETHER?

Twin parents, with babies who often share a room, deal with sleep challenges that a shared sleeping space presents. Some families find that their babies can sleep through each other's cries during the night but can't manage it during naps. Other families find that their babies are woken by each other's noises all the time, and they decide to separate them. The decision to have your twins share a room or not is highly dependent on individual circumstances. In general, when clients come to us with sleep challenges, we often suggest separating their babies temporarily, until the challenge has been worked out. If you are experiencing difficulty with one twin waking the other during a nap, try separating them into different rooms, as far away in the house as possible. But who do you move? Counterintuitive as it may seem, move the twin who isn't currently presenting sleep challenges. Then go to the other baby and work on their sleep in the nursery. You can choose to flip that scenario by letting your easy sleeper take a solid nap in the nursery while you work with the struggling sleeper elsewhere, it's entirely up to you.

NAP ENVIRONMENT AND ROUTINE

We will say it again: *Daytime sleep is a different beast than nighttime sleep.* We don't want you throwing all of the work you have done around nighttime sleep out of the window; we want you to use it to your advantage. Good naps require a great sleeping environment that is cool, dark, and quiet. Abbreviate your bedtime routine during naptime to set the tone that sleep is coming. If you normally change diapers, dim the lights, sing a song, rub their backs, and then throw on the white noise, you should go through those steps (for *both* babies if they are napping separately). We suggest abbreviating your bedtime routine, but don't skimp on it either. The risk is an outcome that isn't what you were hoping for.

SYNCING THE NAP SCHEDULE

Every twin parent's dream is getting their twins to nap *at the same time.* In the spirit of full disclosure, we have to tell you that getting your twins to synchronize their napping schedules is a constant work of art, regardless of how great your sleepers are. The key is laying them down and getting them up from naps at the same time. What if one wakes before the other, you ask? We don't suggest that parents go running to get that baby out of bed, but instead allow them some time to hang and play in their crib. Give them 15 minutes or so and then get *both* babies up from their nap. Remember if one nap is a total bust, save your sanity, evaluate what you need to adjust at the next nap and move on with your day. You can always try again at a later time.

HOW MANY NAPS?

If you continue to struggle with short naps when your babies are seven, eight, or nine months old, you will want to take a look at how long they are staying awake between naps and how many naps they are taking per day. Beyond the first four to six months of age when their sleep rhythms are inconsistent, short naps usually happen due to your babies being overtired. Understanding age-appropriate wakeful windows and managing how many naps your babies are taking per day will help you improve your napping situation. For example, if your eight-month-old is taking three short, crappy naps per day, consider shifting their schedule so they begin taking two naps (the earliest nap starting no earlier than 8:00 a.m.). On the days that naps are terrible and don't seem to work out at all, put your babies to bed early.

Suggested Naps by Age

AGE	WAKEFUL WINDOW	NUMBER OF NAPS PER DAY
Under 2 months	45 minutes to 1 hour	4 or more
3 months	1.5 hours	4
4 to 5 months	2 hours	4 transitioning to 3
6 to 7 months	2.5 hours	3 transitioning to 2
8 to 9 months	3 hours	2
10 to 12 months	3 to 4 hours	2 (transitioning to 1 nap between 12 and 18 months)

Source: BabyCenter.com

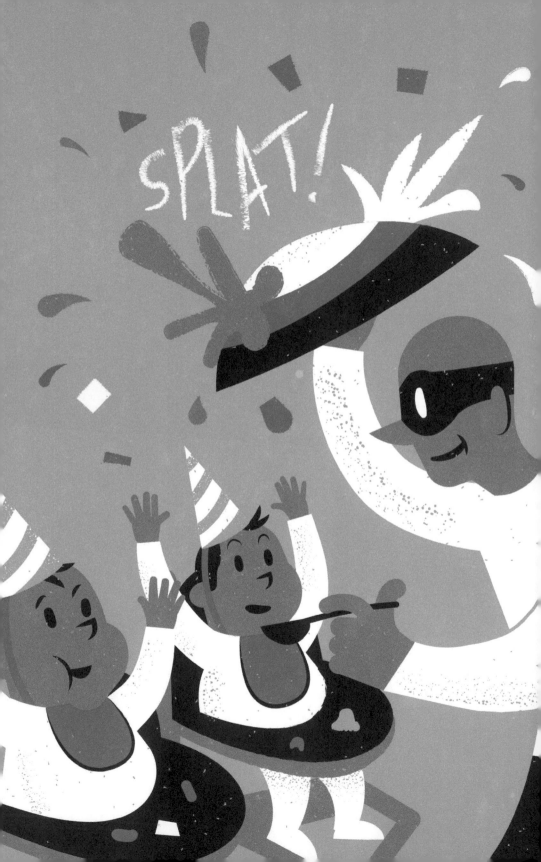

CHAPTER SEVEN
NINE TO TWELVE MONTHS

If you feel like the past nine months have been a blur, you're not wrong. You will never hear a twin parent say that the first year is a breeze. But here you are, nearing the final stretch of this wild and crazy year. You're coming up on a huge parenting milestone and with that will likely come some bittersweet emotions. It is exciting to have outgrown the newborn stage because your sleep is suffering less, your kids are communicating more, and their personalities are flourishing by the day. But now they're on the go, discovering new ways to explore their world, getting into everything, and beginning to team up on you.

Hopefully you've hit your stride. You've probably stopped in your tracks a few times to say things like, "Stop wiping your boogers on your sister!" or "Why are you licking the dog bowl?" or "Where is your brother's diaper?" And if it hasn't happened to you yet, it's coming. With twins, it seems like those moments happen earlier than most because you are constantly keeping *two* babies out of trouble. We'd love to say the chaos slows down, but it just keeps coming. Take it from us, these are the rules to live by. Rule number one: Always be able to adapt. Rule number two: Never forget rule number one.

Milestones

Where has time gone? If you don't already, you will soon understand the saying "The days are long, but the years are short." Your twins are likely mobile, or close to it, learning to crawl, pulling up on things, or even taking those first steps. They are babbling, forming some of their first recognizable words and continually imitating conversations. They may even have teeth! The following milestones as defined by the CDC give you an idea of what to expect at this stage.

SOCIAL AND EMOTIONAL

More and more your babies are beginning to understand their relationship with you, as well as their own autonomy. Now, more than ever, they will begin to assert their personal preferences. When they are told "no," they will understand its meaning but probably won't like it much. They will begin to recognize themselves in a mirror and may cry when you leave the room because they now understand that you are still nearby even when they can't see you, which is why peek-a-boo has probably become their favorite game. With twins, this can be even more fun. Hold up something in between them and yell "Peek-a-boo!" Then take it away and watch them crack up at each other!

VISUAL AND HEARING

Occasionally you will catch your twins communicating with each other in a way that can be hard to describe. Eat those moments up. It's pretty cool to be a bystander while your babies learn to communicate with you, let alone develop a communication style with each other. The babbling will continue as they imitate conversations more and more and, while most of it is unrecognizable, you may get to hear "dada." When you do, prepare for your heart to burst. But lucky you, you get to experience moments like these twice as often.

MOVEMENT AND PHYSICAL DEVELOPMENT

Your twins might look like they are scaling the side of a mountain as they learn to pull up on furniture, stand on their feet (possibly on each other), and even try to take small steps. Some may take off and walk in the coming months. Their hand-eye coordination has tremendously improved, so now they are able to point, pick things up with their fingers and thumbs rather than with their fists, feed themselves (with their hands and utensils), and drink from cups without a spout. Twins tend to do a lot of trading with each other and practice handing things back and forth.

Medical Schedule

While they have slowed down a bit, the well-check appointments occur at 9 months and again at 12 months. Continuing to attend the appointments with the all-hands-on-deck approach is helpful with mobile babies in a doctor's office. Here's what's coming at this stage, as indicated by WhatToExpect.com:

NINE-MONTH VISIT

This will involve a formal developmental screening where your doctor will ask you about your babies' growth and behavior, and observe while you play with them. The intention is to screen for developmental delays by seeing how your babies learn basic skills. If they haven't already, your babies will receive the final dose of hep B and the third dose of IPV.

TWELVE-MONTH VISIT

At this visit, you can expect to get the third or fourth dose of Hib and a fourth dose of PCV between now and 15 months. There will likely be a dose of the measles, mumps, and rubella vaccine (MMR), the varicella vaccine, and one dose of the hepatitis A vaccine between now and

23 months. Your babies will need to get another dose of hepatitis A six months after the first dose. At this appointment your doctor may also perform a lead screening.

Sleeping

Nine months have given you ample time to establish good habits around sleep and set schedules. You might be ready to do the work needed to get your babies sleeping through the night, without feedings, but we understand that the decision to formally sleep train your babies is a deeply personal choice. Ultimately, the goal is to get your babies through the night without needing to eat much before 6:00 a.m. or 7:00 a.m. Here are indicators that the next natural step is weaning the nighttime feeds:

★ Your babies have doubled their birth weight.

★ Their bedtime routine is well established.

★ The sleep environment is just right.

★ Your babies are well versed in being laid down drowsy, but awake.

WEANING NIGHTTIME FEEDS

If your babies are ready to sleep through the night (and so are you), you will want them to consume the calories they usually get from their nighttime feedings during the day. After you've tracked your babies' habits and determined when the night feedings occur (say, 11:00 p.m. and 4:00 a.m.), you should work to eliminate the feeding that occurs earliest in the morning (say, 4:00 a.m.). If your twins are bottle-feeding, reduce the ounces in that bottle by a half ounce every three days. If your partner is breastfeeding, reduce the nursing session by two minutes every three days. Keep this up until that bottle/feeding is completely eliminated and the waking at that hour has stopped fairly consistently, then work in the same way to eliminate the next nighttime feeding (11:00 p.m.). We had great luck with this process as described in Suzy Giordano's book, *Twelve Hours' Sleep by Twelve Weeks Old*.

Remember, you have twins, so it is to be expected that one baby might wean sooner than the other. We do suggest, to save your sanity, that you eliminate one feeding for both babies before you begin working to eliminate the next one.

If your babies wake after you've ditched a feeding, don't revert back. Instead, let them try to get themselves back to sleep by self-soothing. If that doesn't work, gently soothe them with minimal interaction. Eventually, with your supportive consistency, your babies will put themselves back to sleep or not wake at all.

BABIES ADAPTING DIFFERENTLY

Some babies adjust well to these changes, while for others it might take more time to warm up to the idea. Just because one twin takes to sleeping through the night doesn't mean the other will do so right away. Play to their strengths and treat them as individual babies as much as you can. Sure, you can change, feed, and provide basic care for your babies simultaneously to be more efficient, but when it comes to sleep, your babies will probably ride the wave a bit differently. Remember to be patient, celebrate the successes of each sleeper, and know that it will all come in due time.

SLEEP REGRESSION: EIGHT TO TEN MONTHS AND TWELVE MONTHS

As soon as one or both of your babies are sleeping through the night, you will get used to getting more sleep. Then they regress a bit and you'll feel like you've been hit by a truck. Your babies' development changes at a rapid pace. There's a lot going on in their brains as they learn to move and soak up language. When your babies start waking at night or are taking shorter naps, it can take its toll on everyone. As described by Nicole Johnson, founder of The Baby Sleep Site, the 8-to-10-month regression can last anywhere from three to six weeks, which can feel like a lifetime, especially when you have twins who likely won't ease out of the regression at the same time. The 12-month regression, often unnoticed by parents, is usually more nap related and characterized by babies refusing afternoon naps. As with all regressions, offer comfort and support, being careful not to make long-term habits (like rocking or nursing your babies to sleep) a solution for this short phase.

DROPPING NAPS

As soon as the last nap of the day starts to affect bedtime, your twins are having trouble napping, or they suddenly want to have a dance party at 5:00 a.m., you may want to look at dropping a nap. In these age-appropriate windows, dropping naps will take a few short adjustments. Pushing your babies to stay awake a bit longer before a nap and being flexible if an early bedtime is needed, will get you through a nap transition rather quickly.

★ Four to three naps: around four to five months

★ Three to two naps: around six to seven months

★ Two to one nap: around 13 to 17 months

Remember, with twins, one baby may be ready to drop a nap while the other isn't. As frustrating as this may be, the baby that still needs an extra nap will sleep better at night—remember that sleep begets sleep. This phase will likely be short, so get ready to power through a bit with an unsynced nap schedule. Ultimately, parents are happier with well-rested babies than perfect nap schedules.

SEPARATING

If your twins sleep in the same room and continue to wake each other up, it might be time to make a temporary split. Things like sleep regressions can be tough, doubly so when both babies have regressed. Remember, only make small adjustments to get things back on course, and don't let them become long-term habits. Rubbing their backs, patting and shushing while your babies calm, rather than picking them up and rocking, still allows your babies to practice self-soothing in their own sleep space with your intermittent support. Play your cards based on the hand you've been dealt, and separate your twins when needed to get through a sleep regression, nighttime wakings, or nap challenges.

Feeding

It is probably safe to assume that you've had to change your shirt twice between breakfast and lunch a time or two. Feeding twins solid food is an art. You'd better duck and cover after each bite because mealtime with two babies still involves throwing, spitting, and rubbing food all over. Beyond 7 to 10 months, solid foods will begin to provide more nutrition to your babies, which means that they will begin to consume less formula or breast milk. The goal at this point is to have a more traditional eating schedule (three square meals and two snacks) in place by one year. According to *Parents*, here are some helpful guidelines to follow:

★ Around nine months, your babies should have 20 to 28 ounces of formula or nurse every three to four hours, and three meals of solid foods (baby-fist-size portions).

★ Around 10 to 12 months, your babies will likely need 16 to 24 ounces of formula or nurse every four to five hours, and three meals of solid foods (baby-fist-size portions).

HOW TO ENCOURAGE A GOOD EATER

Long gone are the days where you had to sit at the dinner table until you finished your vegetables (or hid them somewhere in the living room). Enforcing the "clean plate rule" likely isn't going to be endorsed by your child's pediatrician, but there are ways to encourage your babies to be healthy, adventurous eaters.

★ **Model healthy eating habits.** The apple doesn't fall far from the tree, so your kids will probably mimic your behaviors around food. Your little eaters are taking an interest in everything you put into your mouth, so practice what you preach the next time you're rolling up to a drive-thru.

★ **Make mealtime family time.** Get into the habit of eating meals as a family from the start. This gives your twins the opportunity to learn mealtime habits from you and sets this routine in place before your kids are older.

★ **Pick your battles.** Yes, as parents, we want our kids to have a diet filled with fruits and vegetables, but battling your kids over food will most likely backfire. Instead, continue to offer a variety of foods (making their plates colorful) and don't make a fuss over things they choose not to eat.

★ **Be creative.** Go beyond the baby basics of peas and carrots and offer a wide variety of foods, even if they are foods you yourself wouldn't eat. Get creative in the kitchen and serve things like salmon, papaya, kiwi, asparagus, or quinoa. If your babies don't care for something, it's not to say they won't like it next Wednesday. Offer rejected foods again and you might be surprised at the tastes that your babies acquire over time.

★ **Avoid processed foods.** No need to start a fad diet tomorrow; however, now is the time to be hyperaware of the ingredients in your food. Why, you ask? Processed foods, full of added salt, sugars, and artificial ingredients, will affect your babies' palates and frankly do not provide the nutrition their growing bodies need. When possible, make homemade versions as often as you can.

Space-Saving Tip: *Lobster claw-style high chairs attach to a countertop, taking up less space than traditional high chairs. The lobster claw chairs are also super easy to disassemble and wash after a messy meal.*

HOW TO INTRODUCE A SIPPY CUP

Crazy as it may seem, babies can start using sippy cups at about the same time they start eating solid foods—as long as they can sit up in a high chair. Babies need to learn that liquids don't only come from boobs or bottles, and the earlier they grasp this concept the better. So as not to overwhelm your babies with so many new adjustments (i.e., introducing solids and a sippy cup simultaneously), allow them some time to acclimate to the idea. Offer a variety of sippy cup brands, filling them with familiar liquids—water, breast milk, or formula—and let your babies take the lead. Our twins really took to the Munchkin Miracle 360°, but many of the choices on the market are great options to try.

HOW TO TRANSITION TO MILK

While we don't want to jump the gun, we do think there is some value in being prepared to tackle new transitions a few months in advance. With the permission of their pediatrician, babies without milk-protein allergies or other health considerations can begin drinking whole milk at one year, even if they continue to breastfeed past their first birthday. Some parents choose to cut out formula cold turkey, while others transition slowly. If you opt for the more gradual approach, you can begin by adding milk into solid foods like oatmeal, cereal, or smoothies. Then add cow's milk (at the same temperature as you typically serve bottles) to formula or breast milk, slowly increasing the ratio of milk in the mixture. Eventually you will be able to serve your toddlers 16 ounces of cold milk each day, as recommended by the American Academy of Pediatrics. One thing to keep in mind as you make this transition is their teeth. Talk to your pediatrician about proper dental care (wiping and rinsing their teeth after meals or milk).

Managing Illness

When your family is slammed with an illness, brace yourself, cross your fingers, and hope it doesn't spread like wildfire. What makes illness tricky with twins is their constant contact; as they take each other's toys and pacifiers it stacks the odds against them. It seems like when one gets sick, they will both be sick, but that is not always the case. Over the years, we've seen our fair share of stomach bugs and viruses, some taking down the entire family, some hitting only the kids, and others infecting just one poor soul. While some of it cannot be controlled, there are ways to prevent, survive, and manage the common childhood illnesses with two. Remember the rule of oxygen masks on an airplane: put yours on first before your babies'. Take precautionary measures while caring for sick kids; you don't want to go down with the ship.

Having sick kids means that you'll be juggling sleepless nights, likely while working, and then coming home after work to help with sick babies again. Having one under the weather is trying enough for families, let alone two at the same time. Remember to take a deep breath and roll with it; life will return to normal shortly.

COMMON ILLNESSES

Preparation and prevention aside, illness will strike at some point. Germs are feisty beasts that will unfortunately find their way into your homes. Having a heads-up about common illnesses can keep you from hitting the panic button the first time your babies come down with the sniffles. According to the CDC, here are some illnesses you may encounter:

★ **Croup.** Croup is caused by a virus targeting the windpipe and voice box, characterized by a barking cough in conjunction with other cold-like symptoms. The barking cough can be managed at night by putting your child in a steam shower for 10 minutes followed by a rush of cold air from the freezer or cold outside air. We always suggest consulting your physician, especially in cases where breathing is affected.

★ **Ear infections.** Ear infections are common in young children, typically occurring in the middle ear from viral and bacterial infections that create pressure between the eardrum and the back of the throat. Most ear infections go away within a few days and are only treated with antibiotics when they are chronic and frequent.

★ **Hand, foot, and mouth disease (Coxsackievirus).** This highly contagious virus is spread through touch, cough, or sneezes. Coxsackievirus typically arises in the summer or fall, and lasts 7 to 10 days. It is characterized by a swollen throat with sores in the mouth and red blisters on the hands and feet.

★ **Pink eye.** Most often caused by a bacterial infection, pink eye is an inflammation of the tissues lining the eyelids, causing redness, yellow discharge, blurry vision, and crusty eyes. It tends to spread like wildfire but can typically be treated with antibiotic drops.

★ **RSV (respiratory syncytial virus).** RSV is an infection of the airways and is most serious in children under two because it can inflame the lungs or cause pneumonia. This is the most common respiratory infection that results in hospitalization in infants, with cold-like symptoms (runny nose, congestion, cough), irritability, and breathing problems.

WHEN TO CALL THE DOCTOR

In general, we follow the theory that it is better to be safe than sorry. After dealing with numerous bouts of croup, ER visits, and doses of steroids, we can say (along with WebMD) that a phone call to the doctor is warranted when you have concerning symptoms.

★ **Dehydration.** When you aren't seeing wet diapers (less than three to four times per day), you are seeing sunken eyes, or your baby is acting lethargic and their mouth is tacky, your child may be dehydrated. A reluctance to eat is important, but dehydration is the more serious concern when a child is sick.

★ **High fever.** Any fever in newborns warrants a call to the pediatrician, but for babies three to six months old, 101 degrees Fahrenheit is your threshold (103 degrees for older children).

* **Preexisting conditions.** If you have a child who has been diagnosed with diabetes, a heart condition, asthma, or other chronic medical conditions, you need to speak with your pediatrician any time they come down with an illness that could compromise their health.

* **Breathing difficulties.** Wheezing, fast or labored breathing, or long pauses between breaths need to be addressed with a medical professional immediately.

MANAGING ILLNESS WITH TWO

Illness with children is inevitable. When it strikes two at a time, there are ways to manage and muscle through.

* **Wash hands like it's going out of style.** Wash your hands like you've never washed before. After touching the keypad at the gas station, pushing grocery carts, handling your cell phone, and then coming home to your babies, the last thing you want to do is touch their faces.

* **When one goes down, separate and designate.** When one twin gets sick, quarantine them to a specific spot in the house, keeping everyone else far away. While this isn't a perfect solution, separating your twins helps contain germs. Also, separate toys, bottles, and lovies. Twins always find a way to share, but while they are sick you want to prevent the passing of germs as much as possible. Tip: Many small plastic toys can be sanitized on the top rack of the dishwasher.

* **Color code *everything*.** Color coding makes twin parenting easier but can be hard to maintain as twins get older. When someone gets sick, tighten up the reins, going back to a strict color-coded routine.

* **Be prepared to waiver.** Twin parents are notorious for their schedules and are willing to do whatever it takes to keep said schedules synced. When it comes to illness, however, be prepared to toss your

schedule aside for a bit. Do whatever is necessary (extra-long naps, etc.) so that your twins' little bodies can fight off the illness and heal.

Jenn: I'll never forget the night my seven-month-old woke up with labored breathing and barking like a seal. It was the most terrifying night we've had as parents to this day, mostly because we had not experienced anything like it before. Immediately, one of us jumped on the phone with our pediatrician while the other called my parents. As soon as we were advised to head to the ER, we threw both boys in the car, dropped the healthy one off with my parents, and went to the hospital. Since this was our first experience with a child in the hospital, we both went for moral support. Infants with labored breathing are a priority. We were treated shortly after arriving and were able to go home first thing in the morning. Since then, we've had three additional ER visits for his croup, but now we have tools to manage when the symptoms arise. Had I known more about common illnesses and strategies to ease their discomfort, that first ER visit might not have been so damn scary.

Making Birthdays Special

Twins share a special bond with their sibling, and a birthday, too. But for young children that can be difficult. Having to split a day where the limelight should be on you, well, it's less than ideal. There are ways to make each of your twins feel special as individuals on their shared day. Remember that birthday celebrations don't have to be extravagant. It's the little touches that will help each of your twins feel unique and special on their birthday.

★ **Birthday posters.** This idea will grow over the years, but it is fun to start while they are young. Create a birthday poster for each baby with a picture from that year. (You'll add more pictures every year.) Then add all of the things that make them unique and special that coincide with their age.

★ **Yes day, all day.** Who doesn't love a day that is all about you? Give each of your kids a day where it's just that, all about them and the only answer to their wishes is YES! Do you want to put chocolate syrup in your cereal? Yes! Ice cream for dinner? Sure! Everyone benefits when they each get a designated day. The wishes don't need to be extravagant, but they should be unique and special to make the day anything but ordinary.

★ **Warm up those pipes.** You never know what your children prefer until you ask them. Do they want "Happy Birthday" sung to them together or separately? Your twins are viewed as a pair for most things in life, making this a quick and easy way for them to feel recognized individually on their birthday.

★ **Date day.** This is something that works well for birthday celebrations but is also a great way to honor your twins individually all year-round. Split your twins up, taking a child on a date day with one parent. Make one-on-one time special and unique, allowing your children to pick their favorite activities.

★ **Love notes.** Finding love notes around the house surely makes our day, which is why we love to hide unexpected (individual) birthday love notes or pictures somewhere in the house, in lunch boxes, or on the bathroom mirrors in dry-erase marker.

★ **Birthday treats.** Not everybody has the same taste, especially when it comes to treats. Even if your twins both love chocolate, for example, it is nice to honor them as individuals by getting them different birthday treats adorned with their name and favorite decor.

Meghan: *When my twins turned one, we were living in my parent's basement while we moved our family to a new city. While other friends around us were throwing elaborate birthday parties for their one-year-olds, I was on a strict budget, living out of suitcases, and trying to adjust to a temporary living situation. Friends would comment, "I'll bet you are throwing a huge party because you have* two!" [or] "I'm sure you can't wait to throw a massive first birthday party for your boys!" And you know what, if I'm being honest, the guilt crept in. Did I want to throw them a party? Sure! But that just wasn't in the cards for us at the time. Instead, we celebrated with close family. There was no elaborate theme, no bells and whistles, just two little cakes that they smashed in their faces and a whole lot of love surrounding not only the boys, but us as well. That first year as a twin parent is something to celebrate. We celebrated all the milestones and the years to come that day. It's not about the birthday flair that is easy to get caught up in. It's about celebrating two awesome boys that have forever changed our lives.

Finally, the Horses' Mouths

Our husbands, Jordan and Matt, have been alongside us as supportive partners, getting their hands dirty while experiencing the journey of twin parenthood. We thought it'd be best to close this book by asking them to share the most important lessons they learned in their first year as twin dads.

> **Matt:** The first year with newborn twins is inevitably trial by fire, especially if these are your first. Prepare yourself for everyone, I mean everyone, to provide you with unsolicited advice. If you're reading this, you're doing what I did and you're looking to get a leg up on the competition . . . that competition being the unknown. Looking back, here are three concepts that really helped me enjoy year one with twins.

> 1. **Oxygen mask.** I was deliberate about reminding my wife to take care of herself first and worked to create opportunities for her to recharge, eat, exercise, etc. I'm not joking when I say there were times when she would have forgotten to eat had I not been there. When necessary, I yelled, "Oxygen mask!" which was the simple reminder for her to take care of herself first knowing that she wouldn't be in any condition to care for our boys.

2. ***Date your partner.*** *It's really easy to allow your relationship to take a back seat. Often, you'll find yourself just trying to get through the next hour, so the idea of planning a date feels like the least important priority. However, planning a date serves multiple purposes. It gives you and your partner something to talk about that doesn't involve diapers or bottles. It gives you something to look forward to, and ultimately the date provides you and your partner the chance to reconnect and recharge as a team, which is what your newborn twins really need—a strong, cohesive team.*

3. ***High fives.*** *Don't underestimate the power of a high five during late-night diaper changing shifts with your partner. Just as you would high-five a teammate who made a key play, you should high-five your partner any time they execute as a great parent, and they should do the same for you. It's a simple but key acknowledgment of their efforts, and it goes a long way in uplifting both parties. Celebrate all the wins, big and small. Embrace the chaos and remember you've got this!*

Jordan: *Being a father is challenging, but it is a priceless and rewarding feat. Babies do not come with owner's manuals, and dads . . . well, we are dads. We are not gifted with the same motherly instincts that mommas have. That being said, it is not an impossible task to raise children. Good news: We can even do it successfully and with swagger. We've got this!*

You will learn early on to embrace the resources available to you, including your partner's. Don't be afraid to ask for help and always have each other's back. Mistakes will be made, but it is all about the recovery and learning how to be successful during the next challenging parenting moment. Teamwork will make the dream work.

Get comfortable with selflessness. This journey is not about you. Yes, you play a vital role, but at times you will have to remove your feelings from the equation. Your job, especially in that first year, is to keep momma and your babies happy and healthy. This can be a daunting task so just keep your head up.

In the early stages of our kids' lives, we are responsible for building the foundation for the individual they will grow and age into. This is a priority to keep in mind at all times even when things are not going exactly as you may have envisioned. My big focus has always been on kindness, love, and humility. Always lead the way with kindness and love. Be unafraid of showing your vulnerable side by embracing your babies with love, lots and lots of love. You will learn, whether it is the easy way or the hard way, that not everything is going to go according to plan. Accept the humility of making mistakes and learning from them. There is not much that I can predict about your parenting journey, but I can guarantee that it will be a wonderfully wild ride.

Baby's First "Guacamole"

Simple and easy

SERVES 6 / PREP TIME: 5 MINUTES / COOK TIME: 1 MINUTE

Avocados make a great starter food for your babies because they are packed full of beneficial nutrients yet are mild in flavor. They are easily digestible and will provide your baby with the healthy fat and carbohydrates that are essential for development.

1 ripe avocado

⅓ can white beans, drained

2 to 3 sprigs fresh basil

Formula, breast milk, or water (if needed)

1. Cut the avocado in half, remove the pit, and scoop the avocado from the skin into the bowl of the food processor or blender.

2. Add the beans and basil to the bowl with the avocado.

3. Purée until smooth, adding small amounts of liquid until the desired consistency is achieved.

Chef's Tip: _Depending on the age of your baby and how much experience they have with solids, you can choose to forgo the food processor/blender and mash the ingredients together. If you go this route, finely chop the basil before adding it into the "guacamole" mixture._

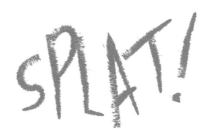

Minty Beet Applesauce

Simple and easy

SERVES 6 / PREP TIME: 10 MINUTES / COOK TIME: 35 MINUTES

This recipe is packed with vitamin C, potassium, antioxidants, and fiber. The flavor is on the sweeter side, but the mint and apple help tone down the rather overpowering flavor of the beets.

2 red beets, peeled and diced into 1-inch pieces

1 apple, peeled, cored, and diced into 1-inch pieces

2 to 3 sprigs fresh mint

Water (optional)

1. In a medium pot, bring a small amount of water to a boil, then insert a steam basket. Steam the beets, covered, for 15 to 20 minutes.

2. Add the apple and steam for an additional 10 minutes.

3. Transfer the steamed ingredients to a food processor. Purée until smooth, adding the mint in at the end. If needed, add small amounts of water until the desired consistency is achieved.

Chef's Tip: *This recipe can be adapted as you work to add more ingredients into your baby's food. It is a hit with or without the apples included!*

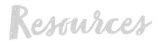

Websites and Blogs

BabyCenter.com. BabyCenter is the world's #1 digital parenting resource. It offers content from health professionals and experts as well as advice from moms and dads. As Parent Contributors to this site, it is one of our favorite parenting resources.

BabySleepSite.com. Started by a mom inspired by her own children's sleep challenges, this site is run by an expert team of sleep consultants. You can find everything from free resources to a members-only library and customized consulting services.

DadsGuideToTwins.com. This site is run by Joe Rawlinson, a twin father, and is a great place for dads to find twin parenting resources and unique support of their own.

Fatherly.com. Fatherly is a great resource for dads, empowering them to raise great kids and lead fulfilling adult lives. The site offers insights to a challenging yet rewarding stage in life.

RaisingMultiples.org. Raising Multiples is the leading national nonprofit provider of support, education, and research on multiple births. They advocate for quality prenatal care and healthy deliveries and supply information to all multiple birth families to support parenting multiples.

TheDad.com. The Dad tells modern day fatherhood like it is. Curated by real dads, the site offers advice and dad jokes.

TwoCameTrue.com. This is our own blog where we share personal stories and write helpful articles aimed at supporting twin families as they navigate life with multiples, from pregnancy to parenting school-aged twins.

WhatToExpect.com. Based on the best-selling *What to Expect When You're Expecting* book series, the site offers medically reviewed health advice on pregnancy and parenting.

References

Amboss. "Multiple Pregnancy." Last modified February 5, 2020. https://www.amboss.com/us/knowledge/Multiple_pregnancy.

American Academy of Pediatrics. "AAP Statement Commending U.S. Consumer Product Safety Commission for Taking Action Against Inclined Sleepers". Date Accessed December 20, 2019. https://www.aap.org/en-us/about-the-aap/aap-press-room/Pages/AAP StatementCPSCInclinedSleepers.aspx

American Academy of Pediatrics. "Car Seats: Information for Families." Last modified February 24, 2020. https://www.healthychildren.org/English/safety-prevention/on-the-go/Pages/Car-Safety-Seats -Information-for-Families.aspx.

American Academy of Pediatrics. "Recommendations for Preventative Pediatric Health Care." Accessed January 7, 2020. https://downloads.aap.org/AAP/PDF/periodicity_schedule.pdf

American College of Obstetrics and Gynecology. "Patient Resources - Multiple Pregnancy: Frequently Asked Questions." Accessed December 10, 2019. https://www.acog.org/patient-resources/faqs/pregnancy/multiple-pregnancy

American College of Obstetrics and Gynecology. "Weight Gain During Pregnancy". Accessed December 13, 2020. https://www.acog.org/clinical/clinical-guidance/committee-opinion/articles/2013/01 /weight-gain-during-pregnancy

American Optometric Association. "Infant Vision: Birth to 24 Months of Age." Accessed January 5, 2020. https://www.aoa.org/patients-and -public/good-vision-throughout-life/childrens-vision/infant-vision -birth-to-24-months-of-age#1.

American Pregnancy Association. "Nutrients and Vitamins for Pregnancy." Last modified October 13, 2019. https://americanpregnancy.org /pregnancy-health/nutrients-vitamins-pregnancy/.

American Pregnancy Association. "Premature Labor." Last modified October 13, 2019. https://americanpregnancy.org/labor-and-birth /premature-labor/.

American Pregnancy Association. "Signs of Labor." Last modified October 13, 2019. https://americanpregnancy.org/labor-and-birth /signs-of-labor/.

The Bump. "Diaper Decisions: Cloth Diapers vs. Disposable." Last modified August 2017. https://www.thebump.com/a/cloth-diapers -vs-disposable.

Canfield, Christie. "Helpful Hints When Introducing Babies and Dogs." American Kennel Club. January 27, 2017. https://www.akc.org /expert-advice/training/how-to-introduce-babies-and-dogs/.

Centers for Disease Control and Prevention. "Important Milestones: Your Baby by Four Months." October 24, 2019. https://www.cdc.gov /ncbddd/actearly/milestones/milestones-4mo.html.

Centers for Disease Control and Prevention. "When, What, and How to Introduce Solid Foods." Last modified October 17, 2019. https:// www.cdc.gov/nutrition/infantandtoddlernutrition/foods-and-drinks /when-to-introduce-solid-foods.html.

Children's Wisconsin. "Birth Defects in Monochorionic Twins." Accessed November 30, 2019. https://chw.org/medical-care/fetal-concerns -center/conditions/infant-complications/birth-defects-in -monochorionic-twin.

Children's Wisconsin. "Postpartum Hemorrhage." Accessed December 1, 2019. https://www.chw.org/medical-care/fetal-concerns-center /conditions/pregnancy-complications/postpartum-hemorrhage.

Choi, Yoonjoung, David Bishai, and Cynthia S. Minkovitz. "Multiple Births Are a Risk Factor for Postpartum Maternal Depressive

Symptoms." *Pediatrics* 123, no. 4 (April 2009): 1147–54. doi:10.1542 /peds.2008-1619.

Ding, Karisa. "How Much Sleep Do Babies and Toddlers Need?" BabyCenter. Accessed February 28, 2020. https://www.babycenter. com/0_how-much-sleep-do-babies-and-toddlers-need_7645.bc.

Ding, Karisa. "Pregnant with Multiples: Nutrition and Fitness Needs." BabyCenter. December 31, 2018. https://www.babycenter.com /0_pregnant-with-multiples-nutrition-and-fitness-needs_3580.bc.

Dolezel, Jodi. "Neonatal Language Terms Used in the NICU." Verywell Family. Last Modified January 18, 2020. https://www.verywellfamily .com/neonatal-lingo-2748438.

Dr. Brown's. "Selecting Your Bottle Nipple Level." Accessed January 18, 2020. https://www.drbrownsbaby.com/selecting-bottle-nipple-level/.

Giordano, Suzy and Lisa Abidin. *Twelve Hours' Sleep By Twelve Weeks Old: a Step By Step Plan For Baby Sleep Success.* New York: TarcherPerigee, 2006.

Good Beginnings/Cedars-Sinai Medical Center. "Glossary of Terms." Accessed December 3, 2019. http://www.goodbeginnings-csmc.org /neonatal/resources/terms.htm.

Gorin, Amy. "Baby's First Foods: How to Introduce Solids." Parents. Accessed January 23, 2020. https://www.parents.com/baby /feeding/solid-foods/starting-solids-guide/.

Her Cottage. "Infant Baby Feeding Chart Schedule and Guide." Accessed January 8, 2020. https://www.hercottage.com /2019/02/02/infant-baby-feeding-chart-schedule-and-guide/.

Hoecker, Jay L. "Is Baby Sign Language Worthwhile?" Mayo Clinic. March 6, 2019. https://www.mayoclinic.org/healthy-lifestyle/infant -and-toddler-health/expert-answers/baby-sign-language/faq -20057980.

Hofmeyr, G., J. F. Barrett, and C. A. Crowther. "Planned Caesarean Section for a Twin Pregnancy." Cochrane. December 19, 2015. https://

www.cochrane.org/CD006553/PREG_planned-caesarean-section-twin
-pregnancy.

Johns Hopkins Medicine. "Twin-to-Twin Transfusion Syndrome (TTTS)."
Accessed November 30, 2019. https://www.hopkinsmedicine.org
/health/conditions-and-diseases/twintotwin-transfusion-syndrome-ttts.

Johnson, Nicole. "How to Survive the 8, 9, or 10 Month Old Baby Sleep
Regression." The Baby Sleep Site. Last modified February 6, 2020.
https://www.babysleepsite.com/baby-sleep-patterns/8-9-10-month
-old-baby-sleep-regression/.

Kelly Mom. "Growth Spurts." Accessed January 10, 2020. https://kellymom
.com/hot-topics/growth-spurts/.

Landau, Elizabeth. "Multiple Births Increase Risk of Postpartum
Depression." CNN. Accessed December 3, 2019. http://www.cnn
.com/2009/HEALTH/03/31/depression.multiple.births/index.html.

March of Dimes. "Getting Ready to Go Home from the NICU." Last
modified June 2017. https://www.marchofdimes.org/complications
/getting-ready-to-go-home-from-the-NICU.aspx.

Mayo Clinic. "Infant Development: Birth to 3 Months." June 29, 2017.
https://www.mayoclinic.org/healthy-lifestyle/infant-and-toddler
-health/in-depth/infant-development/art-20048012.

Mayo Clinic. "Infant Development: Milestones from 10 to 12 Months."
June 27, 2017. https://www.mayoclinic.org/healthy-lifestyle/infant
-and-toddler-health/in-depth/infant-development/art-20047380.

Mayo Clinic. "Postpartum Depression." Accessed December 3, 2019.
https://www.mayoclinic.org/diseases-conditions/postpartum
-depression/symptoms-causes/syc-20376617.

Medical News Today. "What's to Know about Acid Reflux in Infants?"
Accessed January 3, 2020. https://www.medicalnewstoday.com
/articles/315590.php#causes.

Medical News Today. "When to Call A Doctor or Midwife." Accessed January 6, 2020. https://www.medicalnewstoday.com/articles /325872.php#when-to-call-a-doctor-or-midwife.

Murkoff, Heidi. "Twin Delivery." What to Expect. Last modified October 26, 2018. https://www.whattoexpect.com/pregnancy/ask-heidi/twin -delivery.aspx.

National Center for Biotechnology Information. "Nutrition Recommen- dations in Pregnancy and Lactation." Accessed November 29, 2019. https://www.ncbi.nlm.nih.gov/pmc/articles/PMC5104202/.

Pausch, Randy. *The Last Lecture.* New York: Hachette Books, 2008.

Postpartum Depression. "Postpartum Depression in Men." Accessed December 3, 2019. https://www.postpartumdepression.org /postpartum-depression/men/.

Raising Children Network. "Bonding and Attachment: Newborns." Last modified January 6, 2018. https://raisingchildren.net.au/newborns /connecting-communicating/bonding/bonding-newborns.

Sass, Cynthia. "How to Eat When You're Pregnant With Twins, Accord- ing to an RD." Health. February 2, 2017. https://www.health.com /condition/pregnancy/what-to-eat-while-pregnant-with-twins.

Shaw, Gina. "Baby Milestones: 6 to 9 Months." WebMD. Last modified October 4, 2011. https://www.webmd.com/parenting/baby/features /baby-milestones-6-to-9-month#1.

Sleep Advisor. "Family & Sleep." Accessed January 20, 2020. https:// www.sleepadvisor.org/family-sleep/.

Sleep Foundation. "How Your Baby's Sleep Cycle Differs From Your Own." Accessed January 2, 2020. https://www.sleepfoundation.org /articles/how-your-babys-sleep-cycle-differs-your-own.

Stanford Children's Health. "Infant Sleep." Accessed January 20, 2020. https://www.stanfordchildrens.org/en/topic/default?id=infant-sleep -90-P02237.

Treadwell, Ashley. "On-Demand vs. Scheduled Feeding: Which is Best for Baby?" San Diego Breastfeeding Center blog. December 9, 2014. https://www.sdbfc.com/blog/2014/12/9/on-demand-vs-scheduled -feeding-which-is-best-for-baby.

WebMD. "How Often Should You Feed Your Baby?" Last modified July 19, 2019. https://www.webmd.com/parenting/baby/baby-feeding-schedule.

WebMD. "Teething: Symptoms and Remedies." June 25, 2019. https:// www.webmd.com/parenting/baby/teething-symptoms-remedies#1.

Index

twins schedule tracker, 78–79
twin-to-twin transfusion syndrome
    (TTTS), 3, 14
TwinZ Pillow, 22, 75, 81
Two Came True (blog), *viii*
TwoCameTrue.com, 149
type 2 diabetes, 16

U

ultrasound, *viii*, 4, 6, 9, 13, 41

V

vaccines
    four-month visit, 88
    one-month visit, 66
    six-month visit, 88
    two-month visit, 66
varicella vaccine, 131
ventilator, 43
VerywellFamily.com, 40
visual milestones, 64
    nine to twelve months, 130
    six to nine months, 104
    three to six months, 86
    zero to three months, 64
vitamin D, 13

W

water, hydration, 13
wean, 43
WebMD, 106, 139
websites, 149
well-checks, 87, 88, 105, 131
WhatToExpect.com, 14, 88, 131, 149
white noise, 20, 69, 91, 109, 110, 126

Y

You Can Two (Hertzfeldt &
    Bonicelli), *viii*
YouTube
    assembly help, 27
    video management, 76

Z

zero to three months, 63
    doctor visits, 65–66
    documenting memories, 75–76
    doing everything for two, 80–82
    feeding, 70–75
    gift of a schedule, 76–77
    milestones, 64–65
    sleeping, 66–70
zinc, 12

Acknowledgments

Jenn: Thank you, Jordan, my rock and friend, for blessing me with this unwavering partnership that has withstood the test of young love, infertility, and now parenthood. Thank you for standing alongside me on this journey. For jumping right in, learning from our blunders, celebrating our wins, and being my cheerleader through it all. I love you to time and space.

Dominic and Matteo, thank you for teaching me to turn all of my fears, doubts, and worries into strengths that I didn't know I had. Thank you for giving me the role that I am most proud of, being your mother.

To my beloved family, mom, dad, and my dear sister Megan, thank you for surrounding me with the kind of love that makes life meaningful.

And to Meghan, thank you for being my loving friend who has become part of my family.

Meghan: Matt, where do I start? Going to my happy hour with my sister at Andrews was the best decision I ever made. Here we are 13 years later, with a crazy life in Colorado and two boys in tow. Our late-night feedings and double diaper changes have shifted to early-morning pond hockey games and afternoon pit stops to the local Colorado breweries. You've got this dad role dialed in; our boys are incredibly lucky to have you as their father. Living life with you is simply the best (sung in a Tina Turner voice).

To my dad, thanks for always showing up. I know when I was little, you were working your ass off, but no matter what, you were present. Those annual dates to do our taxes and eat at Fuddruckers mattered. No softball game or dance performance was missed. Words cannot repay the love and gratitude I have for you and our relationship. I love you, Dad.

To John, my oldest by three minutes, may you turn 16 and 21 first. You're welcome. To Max, my youngest, remember to tune out your brother, for he thinks he's wiser. You're younger and can get away with anything.

To you both, I want you to know there is nothing I love more than being your mom. From the songs you both get stuck in my head to the pucks in the shins I take as your goalie, I wouldn't change a minute of this life. Not only do you both make me a better person, but you also remind me to pause and appreciate the little things. I love you most!

Mom, thanks for always being my number one fan and encouraging me to do big things and to "take the risk." From jamming out to Cher, crying alongside each other in *Steel Magnolias,* or accidentally wearing camo on the same day, you are one in a million. Love you more!

To my sister, Holly, we'll always have Estes. Thank you for always believing in your little sister and knowing that the Buffs are always going to be better than the Rams. Hair doesn't count. Connie, from Amazon to QVC, with us, no good gadget will go untouched.

To Jenn, holy cow, we pulled this off during the holidays! Cheers to you for taking a risk with me and creating something we thought would only be a dream. You are a great teammate and I value your friendship so much.

Jenn and Meghan: To our Two Came True community, your support continues to amaze us! Thank you for coming along for the ride, sharing your stories with us, and trusting us to be part of your village.

Thank you once again to our fantastic team at Callisto, especially our editor, Mo, for believing that these two moms could be the voices expectant twin dads could learn from.

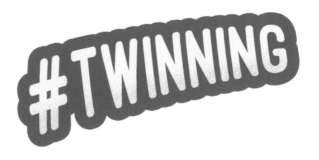

About the Authors

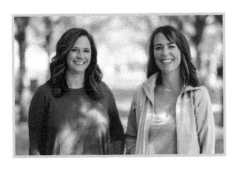

Jennifer Bonicelli and **Meghan Hertzfeldt** are the authors of the book *You Can Two!: The Essential Twins Preparation Guide* and cofounders of TwoCameTrue.com, the popular parenting website, where they blog candidly about life as moms raising multiples—parenting, sleep challenges, and all things in between. Jenn and Meghan have been published online by publications including BabyCenter, Today, Pregnant Chicken, TwinGo Carrier, Multiples Illuminated, and Multiples and More.

Meghan earned her BA in communication from the University of Colorado Boulder and later completed her MAEd in elementary education at Simmons University in Boston. She currently lives in Fort Collins, Colorado, with her husband, Matt, twin sons, John and Max, and black lab, Cash. Their adventures just keep getting better as a family of four.

Jenn, a Colorado native, ventured to Santa Clara University in California to earn a BS in political science and a BA in Spanish. She later returned home to complete her MAEd in curriculum and instruction at the University of Denver. She currently lives in Denver, Colorado, with her husband, Jordan, twin boys, Dominic and Matteo, and their wildly energetic springer, Bella. As a family of four, they are living their best life!

Facebook: Facebook.com/TwoCameTrueBlog

Instagram: Instagram.com/TwoCameTrue

Pinterest: Pinterest.com/TwoCameTrue

Twitter: twitter.com/twocametrue

CPSIA information can be obtained
at www.ICGtesting.com
Printed in the USA
LVHW070420020221
678032LV00023B/4357